It's Not the Strongest That Survives

It's Not the Strongest That Survives

A search for answers in the battle against glandular fever and ME/CFS

Lily Whelan

Copyright © 2024 Lily Whelan

The moral right of the author has been asserted.

Apart from any fair dealing for the purposes of research or private study, or criticism or review, as permitted under the Copyright, Designs and Patents Act 1988, this publication may only be reproduced, stored or transmitted, in any form or by any means, with the prior permission in writing of the publishers, or in the case of reprographic reproduction in accordance with the terms of licences issued by the Copyright Licensing Agency. Enquiries concerning reproduction outside those terms should be sent to the publishers.

The information in this book does not constitute medical advice and is not intended to diagnose, treat, cure, or prevent any condition or disease. Please consult your doctor before making any decisions or changes relating to your health. Neither the publishers nor the author will be held liable or responsible for any loss or damage allegedly arising from any suggestion or information contained in this book. The use of this book implies your acceptance of this disclaimer.

Troubador Publishing Ltd
Unit E2 Airfield Business Park,
Harrison Road, Market Harborough,
Leicestershire. LE16 7UL
Tel: 0116 2792299
Email: books@troubador.co.uk
Web: www.troubador.co.uk

ISBN 978-1-80514-404-5

British Library Cataloguing in Publication Data.
A catalogue record for this book is available from the British Library.

Printed and bound by CPI Group (UK) Ltd, Croydon, CR0 4YY
Typeset in 11pt Minion Pro by Troubador Publishing Ltd, Leicester, UK

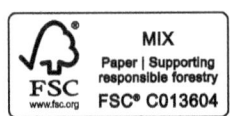

For M & J, for giving me my 'happy ever after'.

This book reflects my recollections as truthfully as memory permits. However, I have made some changes to names and places to protect the privacy of certain people who appear in it. Also, although I have studied science and nutrition, I am not a medic, so you should check with your doctor before embarking on any of the lifestyle changes, or taking any of the medicines or remedies, mentioned in my story. (And while you're checking with your doctor, you might like to recommend this book to them too!) Lily Whelan is a pseudonym.

'According to Darwin's Origin of Species... *it is not the strongest that survives; but... the one that is able best to adapt and adjust to the changing environment in which it finds itself.'*

Professor Leon Megginson

Foreword

Dr. Gavin Spickett

Doctors are required by the General Medical Council to reflect upon their practice. I have been involved in Lily's care for most of my working life as a consultant, so her invitation to read, comment on and finally to provide a foreword is perhaps the ultimate opportunity to reflect on my own practice. Perhaps the most important and humbling perspective for me is that I know so little of the real lives and thoughts of my patients, even those that I have looked after over many years. As a doctor, my interaction with a patient is just like a line touching the circle of life: one tiny point of contact. There is so much that I have not known, although much that I would have suspected or predicted.

Lily told me quite a few years ago that she intended to write her story and I have encouraged her to do so. Indeed, I had told her she had to complete it before I retired, which she did! She has produced an eloquent picture of what it is like for someone to be struck down with a chronic and severely debilitating illness that has turned her life upside down. Her greatest ambition was to be a leading scientist, and it has been very hard for her to accept that her illness has prevented her from achieving this. This book is about how she has managed to come to terms with her illness and its effect on her life and arrive at a place where she is comfortable with who she is, comfortable with her family, her parents, her husband and her son.

I read this book with some trepidation, having been forewarned that she would mention me. When she gave me the draft to read at one of her clinic appointments, I randomly opened it and it fell open at a page where she was describing one of her visits to my clinic, at which point she threatened to take it away again if I read it in front of her! It has been an irresistible read that moves on apace. There is a gentle humour that pervades the book even at the bleakest of times. Her illness has tested both her and her family in many ways.

Her fascination with science shines through. She has always wanted to understand the science behind her illness and this made for some interesting discussions when she has visited the clinic. People with long-term illness require a framework in which they can manage their illness, which is based on knowledge and understanding. It is easier to cope when you understand what the illness is. Doctors should play a role as a guide in this journey of self-discovery. At times her frustration with the lack of research into CFS/ME would bubble over. The appearance of long Covid during the coronavirus pandemic has at last kick-started meaningful research into what causes persistent illness in some individuals after viral infections, not just coronaviruses but also once again EBV. EBV has been a suspect for over sixty years!

Lily has documented her journey and it will be valuable to anyone else struggling to make sense of long-term illness. However, it is not just a self-help guide. I have learnt from it and I hope readers will also find something that will help them in the trials of life.

Dr. Gavin Spickett
Author of the *Oxford Handbook of Clinical Immunology and Allergy.*

Prologue

I only nipped into Boots to pick up my tablets, but I came away having made a life-altering decision.

I remember standing behind a student in a queue for the tills, hoping the guy would pay quickly. My face was swelling up again, and my zombie brain fog had returned. I needed to get home *now*. But as the student handed over a fiver to the smiley cashier, she asked if he had a points card. 'Or would you like one?' she chirped, probably for the eighty-sixth time that day.

No way did I want to hang around while he tried to remember his first pet's name. It was time to practise my Jedi mind-control skills on him. *No, you don't want one*, I urged the back of his head.

He wanted the card, of course. What were the odds? The cashier did a double take, evidently thinking she'd misheard him. Afterwards, she took a distinct liking to him – even offered to help him fill in the form. Soon they were laughing and flirting so much, I thought I'd stumbled onto the set of the latest romcom. As the student boomed out his personal details, I glanced around to check there were no criminals lurking behind the shampoos, recording his sensitive data.

As you do.

Then he said something that made my breath catch: his date of birth. He was born in October 1994. That was the exact month and year that my life changed forever – when I first contracted my illness. I looked at him again. He was a strapping lad, all stubble and muscle. Judging by his Durham University hoody, he had probably been out rowing that morning. How was it possible that someone could be born and grow up in the time that I had been ill? And why was society, not to mention the medical profession, still as confused about my illness now as it had been all those years ago?

That was the moment I knew I had to get this book out.

Health organisations have estimated that there are seventeen million people worldwide with my disability. And that was *before* the world was hit by coronavirus. This is a mind-boggling figure for an illness that the Canadian ME/CFS Consensus reportedly described as being more debilitating than most other medical problems in the world, including chemotherapy and HIV. Just stop and think about that for a moment. More debilitating than chemotherapy and HIV.

So, what is this illness?

That's just the trouble; no one really knows. It doesn't even have a name that everyone can agree on. Myalgic Encephalomyelitis (ME) is the title most people will be familiar with. Strictly speaking, though, Myalgic Encephalomyelitis means 'inflammation of the brain and spinal cord with muscle symptoms'. Whereas doctors say sufferers don't actually have inflammation of the brain and spinal cord.

So, what other names are there? In 2015, the National Academy of Medicine (formerly the Institute of Medicine) in the US suggested calling the illness SEID, or Systemic Exertion Intolerance Disease. Catchy, I know. Other titles include Chronic Fatigue Syndrome (CFS), Post-Viral Fatigue Syndrome (PVFS), Chronic Fatigue Immune Deficiency Syndrome (CFIDS)… the list goes on. The problem with those names is the use of that common word 'fatigue'. Many patients and clinicians don't like it because its inclusion trivialises the condition and leads to stigmatisation. We are not tired. We are *ill*.

The mislabelling of the condition has been a major factor in its misconception. It has helped to perpetuate the myth that ME/CFS (or whatever name you prefer) is not a physical illness but a psychological one. This is an absurd thing to suggest. Yet, even some doctors think that ME/CFS is a disease of psychosocial origin. Perhaps that is understandable when you consider that, at the time of writing this, less than a third of medical school curricula, and less than half of medical textbooks, include *any* information on the condition. Stephanie Munn, a London consultant who suffered with the illness for four years, reported in the British Medical Journal (BMJ) that she 'witnessed colleagues making appalling generalisations about people with ME'.[a] One of my immunologists likened the response to the illness from some doctors as 'no different from racism, or homophobia, or any other prejudice.'

Are times changing? In 2019, the House of Commons passed a resolution calling on the Government to provide increased funding for biomedical research into ME/CFS. Then coronavirus rampaged across the globe, leaving in its wake millions of people with post-viral fatigue. 'NHS faces post-coronavirus tsunami as survivors are struck down by ME',[b] headlined *The Sun* newspaper. The BMJ agreed: 'Patients with chronic fatigue are likely to present in increased numbers to all forms of medical practice worldwide... [It] must not go unrecognised'.[c]

It must not go unrecognised, no. Nor must it be played down nor misunderstood any longer. That is why I am telling my story.

I fell ill in October 1994. It has taken well over twenty years to turn my life around, as well as hundreds of blood tests and enough antiviral drugs to start my own pharmacy. In that time, I have grappled with a legion of sceptical doctors and dabbled with alternative therapies. I have lost friends, worn out my tear ducts, and been forced to sacrifice all hope of pursuing the career I so desperately wanted. But I have also found strength and understanding, and developed a sense of humour that anyone with this illness will need if they are going to endure it.

Writing this was hard, and I don't just mean from a physical perspective. Once my experiences started spilling out onto the page, I began having nightmares. You know the ones where you're naked in front of fully clothed people? Or is that just me? I realised how tight-lipped (and at times dishonest) I had been with friends and family concerning my ill health. As I relived my memories, I found myself alternately laughing, crying and cringing at my younger self.

Yet I feel blessed to have been able to write this. Most people who have my condition do not have the health to make their voices heard. So please excuse the blinkered girl at the start of my story. She really has learnt a lot by the end.

My hope is that a few of my readers will have done so too.

Chapter 1

It all started with a ski trip, and a run-in with one of the cool crowd at school. I was in the common room one Monday evening when Gertie announced that the ski team was a member short. If anyone was able to ski, could they let her know? I thought I'd give it a go. Wouldn't want to let the school down, and who knew, it might be fun. So, I walked over to Gertie, parting the sea of clones around her, and told her I'd do it.

She was clearly surprised because she looked me up and down and said, 'You do actually have to be *good*, you know.'

I guess I didn't look trendy enough to be a skier. According to the boys, I was officially one of the 'nice girls' (it didn't have the kudos of the babes or athletes, but I was happy to take it), so I said, 'Look, if it's a giant slalom, I'll be fine. I've done them before.'

'Competitive skiing isn't like skiing with Mummy and Daddy,' said Gertie. 'But if you want to see if you're up to it, we're going to the dry ski slope on Wednesday night.'

Gertie didn't know that I had been skiing since I was in nappies. Most kids get dragged down to Clarks for their first shoes, but the earliest footwear I remember wearing was ski boots. My parents were both keen skiers so, while I was still a toddler, my name got added to their Weardale Ski Club membership. On any weekend when there was more than a dusting of snow, my dad drove us over to the Pennines where I honed my slalom skills by dodging the rocks and heather poking through the slush.

Growing up, I had few concerns beyond which of my family's fruit trees I would sit under to make daisy chains. I had loving parents and an elder brother who teased me only once every other day. Don't get me wrong, I had duties as daughter of the family; I had to look after the dog, and keep my room tidy, and hand around nibbles at the occasional dinner party. And whenever my brother appeared in his battered cowboy hat needing someone to kill, I would have my own cowboy hat on before his plastic gun was out of its holster.

There was no doubt, though, that I was different from the rest of my family. I lacked the competitive streak that seemed to run through the others. Once, aged seven at a school sports day, I slowed down from leading the Class Four sprint so I could cross the finishing line holding hands with my friends. My dad tried for years to instil some ambition in me, but I just viewed school as an extension to my social life.

That changed in my final year at primary school. The teacher took delight in picking on one pupil in each class, and I was her latest victim. My mum complained, but nothing changed, so I hardened myself to the teacher's taunts of how stupid I was and just got on with it. Anyway, when I started secondary school, I was determined to be successful if only to prove the witch wrong. Then pubescent hormones came into play, and, before I knew it, I was as competitive as the next girl. But my real drive came only when I found science.

Look at the pompous way I wrote that – as if I'd said I had found God or something. But it did feel like a road-to-Damascus moment when, aged eleven, I sat on a stool in my first chemistry lesson. It wasn't the theatrical explosions that appealed to me, or the puffs of coloured smoke wafting around the laboratory. OK, not *just* those things. It was the fact that, with science, it seemed like you could solve everything. This was the '90s, when scientists were working on the Human Genome Project and cloning a sheep. I desperately wanted to be part of that scene. With a top job in science, I thought I'd be able to change the world.

So, I swotted and smiled my way through early adolescence, convinced that my future was mapped out like a flow chart. I didn't realise there is so much that *can't* be predicted or explained. Nor did I have any idea that I was about to be hit with an illness that nobody understood.

Fast forward six years from that first science lesson. I was now in the sixth form of a new school and within touching distance of the Big Dream. I had been invited for interview for the Natural Sciences course at the University of Cambridge. My school was great in that it encouraged you to have a go at everything, from community service to music competitions. As children, we are led to believe we can achieve anything if we put our minds to it. But people forget that the body has to be on board too.

Which brings me back to that trip to the dry ski slope. Truth be told, by the time Wednesday came around I wasn't in the mood for skiing. I had been feeling nauseous all day, a bit... spaced out. But I shrugged it off as nothing because I never got ill. Even colds were things that happened to other people. Besides, I had something to prove to Gertie after the way she had dismissed me.

So, that evening, I found myself in the school minibus on the way to the dry ski slope. Gertie was there, along with the rest of the ski team and our teacher, Mr Arnold. I still had that feeling of queasy detachment. If anything, it was getting worse, but I kept telling myself that I did *not* feel sick and my head *was* still attached to my body. When we arrived at the slope, I kitted up and flitted down the course.

'Looks like we have a new star skier!' said Mr Arnold. Although he tempered his enthusiasm after he saw Gertie's face.

The 'star' bit was a stretch, but I didn't say anything. I was just excited that I now had the British Schools' Dry Slope Championships to look forward to, as well as my Cambridge interviews.

Life was such fun.

*

The next day, my mum – a consultant psychiatrist – said I looked disturbingly pale. She sent me to the GP for blood tests, thinking I might have glandular fever. Glandular fever is sometimes called 'the kissing disease', so there must have been a serious outbreak of snogging at my school because the illness was rife at that time.

All my tests came back negative. That should have been good news. My parents, though, could see that something was wrong, and deep down I knew it too. As my symptoms lingered, I became practised at brushing off other people's concerns. A few days before I was due to compete in the national ski finals, I was walking across a courtyard at school, smiling at a butterfly, when Mr Arnold stopped me. The sun reflecting off his glasses dazzled me.

'Lily,' he said. 'Can I have a word?'

'Yes, sir,' I replied. (I was a cringe-worthily polite and eager student.)

'The ski finals are this weekend, and I know you haven't been well.'

'I'm OK.'

'Are you?' Mr Arnold pushed his glasses up the bridge of his nose. 'I heard you might have glandular fever. You mustn't feel you *have to* compete on Saturday. What matters is your health.'

'I'm fine, sir, really.' And I gave him my cheesiest smile to convince him – or to convince myself, perhaps.

In the lead up to the competition, I had found it increasingly difficult to get out of bed each morning. On the day itself, my head felt like mud, and it took every scrap of willpower to coax my body into first gear. I caught a lift into school and hauled myself onto the minibus, then dozed all the way to the dry ski slopes in Sheffield.

Once there, the adrenaline kicked in. Through the minibus window I saw teenagers milling about. There was a hum of chatter broken occasionally by a commentator's voice booming over the Tannoy. The other schools' competitors looked so professional in their team fleeces and helmets. Whereas we had turned up in jeans and puffer jackets.

I gazed at the dry ski slopes. Competitors were already streaking down the giant slalom course, while on a second slope beside it, more skiers were gliding down in groups, showing off their jumps and turns.

'It's *so* cool!' I whispered.

Mr Arnold slid open the side door of the minibus for us to climb out. 'Now, you'll all get a practice run before the competition,' he said, 'but we have to wait our turn. So, you can either stay here or—'

I was already gone. I headed towards the action, desperate to get a closer look at this fantasy world for skiers.

Some of the boys came with me, and we passed the main building with its public viewing space to form a row at the bottom of the slalom. There was a crowd of students applauding each skier as they skidded to a halt. The commentator kept up a constant stream of announcements, but I wasn't listening; I was sussing out the talent.

Before I knew it, it was my turn to compete. I took the ski lift to the top of the slalom and moved into position, shins pressed against the gate, ready to go. At the bottom of the course, the spectators were no more than clusters of specks. Then… *Beep*… I was off!

I flew around the first post, the second, and as I approached the third it occurred to me that I might collapse. My vision clouded. It was like I was seeing the world through a pane of glass. *Keep going*, I thought. *Keep going.* For the merest second, I felt my left ski begin to slip away from me. Then the muscles in both legs started to tremble. But I forced myself to continue, left, right, left, right, and soon I was flying through the finishing posts.

People rushed towards me. I was vaguely aware of pats and hugs from the boys, but I was concentrating so hard on staying upright that the rest was a bit of a blur.

'Are you OK?' someone asked.

'Of course,' I said through my daze. 'I just need…'

What? What did I need? A doctor? A hospital?

'I just need a Twix,' I said, clicking out of my skis and stumbling towards the vending machines. At that age, there were few problems in life that couldn't be solved with chocolate.

We didn't find out our rankings on the day because we left the ski slope early. But back at school the following Monday, Mr Arnold informed me I'd come fifth in my category. I wondered if they'd made a mistake with the timings but was too busy enjoying the moment to question it.

Later, when I was bored in maths class (because I was *never* bored in chemistry or biology), I stared out of the window and watched the birds peck for crumbs while I dreamt of my future. I was going to be a skier – you know, when I wasn't discovering the meaning of life. I could fit the skiing in when I needed some fresh air to keep the brain cells working. I had it all planned. I would go to the University of Cambridge and join their ski team and…

Well, I wasn't sure about that last 'and' because you never know exactly what's around the corner.

It was probably just as well that I didn't.

*

When I woke up the next morning, I could hardly open my eyes. I had to peer through slits. Tingly aches rippled along my legs. I called for my mum, but my voice was so hoarse she didn't hear me. I felt trapped. Eventually, I managed to haul myself out of bed and stagger to my mirror. A stranger looked back at me: a girl with a face as round as a pufferfish. My eyelids were so swollen that the groove of the socket had almost disappeared.

When my mum came to check on me, she saw me and rushed over.

'Let me examine you,' she said, taking my pulse. Then she stuck a thermometer under my tongue, prodded and poked in a doctor-like fashion. She looked stumped. 'I thought it was glandular fever,' she explained. 'But I can't feel enlarged glands. We'd better get you to the GP.'

I had to go somewhere? I didn't think I was capable even of getting dressed, but eventually, with Mum's help, I pulled on some clothes. Then my dad drove us to the surgery. I felt so detached it was like watching my life on a television screen. I stretched out on the back seat and thought, *this is serious*. And for a moment it occurred to me that I might have more important issues to deal with than getting into Cambridge.

The doctor's surgery was a brown-beige room of gloom filled with pensioners flicking through yellowing magazines. I was soon called in by a bright and inquisitive GP. That was such a godsend, because when you feel like you're fighting for your life, you don't want one of those haven't-got-a-clue doctors. She gave me the once-over, then said, 'It's glandular fever.' Considering how ill I felt, she looked unreasonably pleased with herself.

'But I couldn't feel enlarged glands,' said my mum.

'There are *chains* of them!'

Suddenly, I was a prop in a med school lecture as the GP showed Mum exactly where to feel. My mother had mistakenly thought that the enlarged glands would be under my chin and down the front of my neck, whereas, in reality, they were down the back of my neck. (I have had my glands felt by a couple of dozen doctors over the years, and all of them, except my immunologists, have made the same mistake.)

'Goodness me!' said Mum, when she found the right areas. 'It's like strings of pearls!'

'I know,' the GP replied, and the two of them grinned at each other, lost in their little doctor world.

'Er, I'm still here,' I croaked.

'We'd better take some blood,' said the GP. 'And do you think you could provide a urine sample?'

Sounded simple enough. But when the doctor waved one of those clear plastic bottles in front of me, it was like a wand casting a lock spell on my bladder. After a few frustrating minutes in the toilet, I staggered back into the waiting room and told my parents it was a no go.

'It's important,' protested Mum. 'They need the urine to check your kidney function.'

'If I can't go, I can't go!' I said. 'What am I supposed to do?'

The pensioners in the waiting room did the tennis eyes between us. The tick-tock of the receptionists' clock was the only sound – until my dad piped up: 'I know, I'll sing to her!'

This was so typical of my father. He thinks there is a song to fit every woe.

So, just when I thought I couldn't get more embarrassed, Dad broke into 'Singin' in the Rain' and other water-based songs, interspersed with splashing sounds. Everyone in the waiting room thought it was hilarious. Or rather, everyone *else* in the waiting room did. I, on the other hand, was mortified. I was seventeen years old and still liked to think I had street cred (hard to believe considering my geekiness, I know).

Then again, the stress of the situation left my bladder bursting, so I guess Dad achieved his aim.

*

When the blood test came back, it confirmed glandular fever. (My earlier blood test must have been a false negative, as can happen when the test is carried out too early in the illness.) It seems crazy to think so now, but when I heard the diagnosis, I was relieved. Finally, I had an explanation for the weird stuff I was feeling. Plus, it was *only* glandular fever. *Hurray!*

At work, Mum started finding out more about the illness. When she came home, she sat on the edge of my bed and waved some pages at me that she'd photocopied from a medical textbook.

'You know you've been feeling like you're looking at everyone through a TV screen?' she said. 'That's called "depersonalisation". Some people get it with the illness. Also, your eyes – the puffiness – that's called "periorbital oedema". Some people get that too.'

Hearing this made me feel a lot better. The monsters under the bed aren't half as scary when you can put a name to them.

Unfortunately, it was a little too soon to break out the bunting. One day, when I had the house to myself, I studied my blood test results more closely. I had learnt that in most glandular fever cases, the level of atypical monocytes – they are like corrupted immune cells – in the blood was about ten per cent. Only in a very severe case would it rise to fifty. Mine was eighty-three.

I wouldn't think about that, though. Instead, I focused on the fact that people typically recovered from the illness in three to six months – the medical book said so, so it must be true. When I look back at that now, I shudder. I wanted to be a scientist, yet here I was carrying out one of the cardinal sins of research: cherry-picking facts to support the conclusion I wanted to reach.

The weeks that followed passed in a virus-tinged blur. I was off school, lying in bed, living off yoghurt drinks since I couldn't get solids down my inflamed throat. I still felt detached from my body, though the nausea would often surface to remind me we remained connected. I lost weight. I was too ill to read or even talk much. And anyone who knows me understands how sick I must be for that to happen. So instead, I spent every minute of every day… thinking.

Glandular fever marked the start of my becoming the person I am today. Up to that point, life had been so easy, but this illness brought everything to a grinding halt. Now, I was alone in an empty house while my friends were at school, my parents were at work, and the world carried on as normal. Just opening my eyes was a challenge. Forcing my body upright felt like torture. For the first time, I began to wonder about people who were struggling. While I had been skipping through life, how many others had been wading through it?

After a few weeks of getting to know my ceiling intimately, I'd improved enough to be able to press the play button on life again. At that time, the medical consensus was that glandular fever sufferers should 'push' themselves back to health as soon as they could. So, one Monday morning, I dragged myself into school. I couldn't take part in sports in case my spleen ruptured (glandular fever often causes a sufferer's spleen to become enlarged). But I threw myself into my studies, rejoined the school orchestra, even scaled the ninety-eight steps up the hill to chapel each morning.

I lasted a week. By Friday, I felt like death. After spending the following weekend in bed, I decided on a new plan of action: I would concentrate on my lessons and cut out all socialising and extracurricular activities. I didn't really mind missing out on those things because I enjoyed science so much. I was also under the illusion that my friends would stand by me when I needed them – and some of them did.

However, many of them started to drift away. Worse, they turned not just their backs on me but also their tongues. I became the butt of jokes and rumours. Some people said that I wasn't suffering from glandular fever but from anorexia (this from a girl who was herself anorexic). Or that I was skiving to avoid an ex (not my style at all). Or that I had turned myself into a hermit so I could spend all my time revising for my upcoming Cambridge interviews (if only!).

The injustice stung. At home I would think, *what can I do to prove how ill I am? And why do I need to prove it at all?* Anyone with sense could see I was struggling. I was only able to get to a quarter of my lessons. Some days I would haul myself into the first class of the day, only to feel so dreadful I had to ring my mum and ask her to collect me at lunchtime.

Back home, I would go straight to bed and *will* my body

to be better for the next day – as if willpower alone could cure me. I knew I was far sicker than my classmates realised. Yet, even I didn't appreciate how ill I really was.

Chapter 2

My Cambridge interviews came around quickly. I had bought my train ticket long in advance, thinking I would be well enough to travel to Cambridge alone. When I wasn't, my dad volunteered to drive me down instead, and I accepted the offer with reluctant gratitude. Then Mum decided to come along so she and Dad could see the city while I was being interviewed. It wasn't the ideal scenario – my personal adventure was being turned into a family outing.

As I climbed into the car that day, I still felt depersonalised – not quite at the watching-the-world-on-TV stage but battling through a mental fog all the same. Because of this, I managed to forget to take any cassettes for my Walkman. All I had was the tape already in the player: the single 'Nothing Compares 2 U' by Sinead O'Connor. I listened to it on repeat for the whole four-hour journey. By the end, it had become my 'Cambridge song'. I felt that nothing in my life compared with how much I wanted to get into the University of Cambridge. Now I am sorry I made that link because for years afterwards, whenever I heard the song, it reminded me of that moment and all that followed after.

The University of Cambridge is composed of thirty-one colleges, but my favourite was Trinity Hall. I had fallen in love with it on a trip to Cambridge the previous year. Each college had its own personality, and after visiting a handful, I had to prioritise between academic reputation, architectural beauty and people. I have never admitted this to anyone before, but I wanted a college with history that was ranked high in science and friendly types. The first time I had walked into the courtyard of Trinity Hall, I was greeted by the welcoming faces of students who were as unpretentious as they were ambitious. I felt like I'd come home.

Now, sitting outside the room where I would be called for my first interview, I was flushed and giddy. When the college tutor – the don – poked his head out and called my name, I positively bounced in. I still get flashbacks from that day: calculating the dimensions of a mitochondrion from an electron micrograph, chatting with a don about what I considered to be the most important scientific discovery ever made… I was in heaven. Of course, I knew the stakes were high, which made me pick my words carefully, but apart from that – nerd alert! – these were the sorts of things I'd have happily talked about all day.

Much later, I found out that when the dons discussed the students they had interviewed, they referred to me as 'the smiley one'. I like that. So much better than 'the pale, blobby one', which would have been just as apt in view of my swollen face.

After my interviews, I left Trinity Hall and walked down an alley to where my parents were waiting in the car. I climbed into the back, stretched out my legs and shut my eyes. My limbs were ablaze with aches.

'Well?' asked my dad.

'Ian!' protested Mum. 'Let her catch her breath. She looks wiped out.'

'She can at least give us the condensed version. Could you answer all the questions, love?'

'Yes,' I replied.

'What about the dons? Were they nice? Did you feel that you clicked with them?'

'Yes,' I repeated, opening my eyes. Then I added wistfully: 'In fact, I want their job.'

In the rear-view mirror, I saw Dad beaming. 'And did you smile?' he asked. 'Were you, you know, your lovely, chatty self?'

'I suppose,' I said, suppressing a giggle.

'Well, then. You're in!'

'Ian!' said Mum again. 'Don't get the poor girl's hopes up.' She was right to be cautious, too. The dons were interviewing three people for every place available. 'Get some rest,' Mum instructed. 'You look a lot blobbier than you did this morning.'

I didn't care because I was still riding an emotional high. I had performed my best despite my illness. The rest was down to fate. I switched on my Walkman and listened to 'Nothing Compares 2 U' all the way back to Durham.

*

The following week, I returned to school. If I was offered a place at Trinity Hall, I would need to get three A grades in my A levels, so I tried to block out my illness and soldier on.

It wasn't enough. My health was slipping, and so were my standards. One time, in biology class, we had to dissect rats.

Being an animal lover, this would have been enough to upset me at the best of times, and of course the boys delighted in telling me how they had seen the animals happily playing in their cages that morning. When the lesson began, we were each handed a rat, stiff with rigor mortis. I got to work, securing its body to my wooden board, little belly upwards, a pin through each paw. I felt sorry for the poor thing, but my head overruled my heart – as it did in those days – and I reminded myself that the sooner I finished the dissection, the sooner I could find somewhere to lie down.

Clutching my scalpel, I made the first incision.

After a while, the ever-present fog in my head began to thicken, and my hands felt like they were on a time lag. *Focus!* I told myself. I'd pinned back the rat's skin and labelled most of the organs already, but I still had the nether regions to dissect. The scalpel in my hand wavered. Not concentrating, I somehow contrived to slice off – and the men among you may want to look away now – the rat's meat and two veg.

Gush! Fluids everywhere.

I went cold all over. The mark for this practical would count towards my A level grade, but more importantly, it was something the other students would never let me live down. Fortunately, they were so engrossed in their work, they didn't notice what I had done. So, I slunk over to the sink and pulled some paper towels from the dispenser. Then I casually began mopping up the mess from my board. Nothing to see here, move along.

'Three minutes left!' shouted the teacher.

I arranged the 'package' as best I could to one side of the rat and wrote my labels. 'Penis', 'Vas Deferens', 'Epididymis'…

When the teacher came around to mark our efforts, she said, 'Right, Lily. Liver, pancreas… Oh!' She chuckled, first quietly, then louder. 'Watch out, boys! Lily's got a knife in her hand and she means business!'

There was a screech of stool legs on tiles as the other students got up to see what had happened.

'Er, I kind of accidentally castrated it,' I said. 'I mean, I was just cutting through the scrotal sac when my hand slipped, and…' But the more I tried to explain, the more I blushed, and the more everyone else laughed.

I made another blunder during a botany practical later that week. It involved an hour and a half of staining microscopic pond life with ink, then studying it under a microscope. You're probably yawning already, but to me, seeing those twitchy microscopic dudes dart about in the petri dish was like being privy to a secret underwater world. As the other students handed in their work and left the laboratory, I was still putting the final touches to my diagrams. I had stumbled through the entire experiment with a brain fog, and I felt elated to be emerging from the lesson unscathed.

Then it happened.

As I turned to see where I had left the open ink jar, my elbow caught it and knocked it over. Black ink rushed across the bench and over my pages of meticulous writing. An hour and a half's work ruined in as many seconds. Horrified, I grabbed the pages and walked to the front of the class.

The teacher, Mr Buckett, was sitting at his desk, humming while he marked. He wore a tweed jacket, breeches and the thick-framed spectacles that earned him the nickname 'Biggles'.

I held up the pages and tried to speak, but all I could muster was a pathetic, 'Sir?'

Mr Buckett looked up, saw my stricken face and the dripping pages. A flash of shock, then he said, 'Thank you, Lily. Another experiment excellently executed.' He reached across his desk and eased my work out of my hand. He was trying so hard not to look at me or the pages, I wondered if he had actually noticed the ink.

'But, sir! They're ruined!'

'I don't see anything ruined.'

Had he lost the plot? 'They're covered in ink!' I said.

'I see no ink,' he replied. Which was impressive considering how much of the stuff had dripped onto the work he was marking. He leant back and placed my assignment in the bin behind him. The ink from my pages immediately stained the wet paper towels inside it. I tasted the saltiness of a tear running down my lips and searched through my blazer pockets for a tissue.

'Lily,' Mr Buckett said. 'It's not important. Go home, get well. Please.'

I'm still grateful to this day for Mr Buckett's kindness. There are so many ways a teacher could have reacted in that situation, but he played it like a pro. In fact, all my science teachers were incredibly kind to me throughout my illness. They seemed to understand what I was going through and were eager to help me in whatever way they could. Their support compensated for some of the pupils' doubts in me.

But whilst it might not have mattered to Mr Buckett what had happened to my experiment, it mattered to me. This was about more than just one ruined assignment; this was another example of my brain fog throwing obstacles in my way. I could ignore the aches and sore throat to get myself into my experiments, but I couldn't stay alert for their duration. For all my resolve, I was losing my way.

I wasn't about to give in, though. The virus might have won a battle, but I wouldn't concede the war. If a tiny parasite, devoid of nucleus, thought it could keep *me* down it had another thing coming. My A levels were later this year, and I would be fully better for them.

So there.

*

Opening my acceptance letter from Trinity Hall was one of the happiest moments of my life. The knowledge that I had gained a place where I most wanted to be – that is something I will carry with me always. On the other hand, it made me push myself even harder to get the grades I needed.

My life settled into a demoralising pattern. Each morning, I would wake up and try to drag myself into school. Even when I managed it, though, I would usually only last a lesson or two before the aches, nausea and fever forced me home again. Then I would be off for another week, alone in the silence of what I was coming to consider as my sick house. Sometimes Holly, my bearded collie, would lie on the carpet alongside my bed and give my hand a lick when it dangled beside her.

Thoughts of Cambridge got me through. I remembered walking down King's Parade in the sunshine and watching the students fly past on their bikes. I wanted so much to be one of them. But the virus had other ideas. One morning at school, I was trying to copy up some work I had missed, only to discover I couldn't write. My pen was poised, but my brain fog was so thick I couldn't find a way through it. *Come on, Lily*, I thought. *It's just copying, for heaven's sake!* But my body was crying out 'stop' so loudly, I couldn't overrule it.

Perhaps I just needed a break – a walk up and down the road to clear my mind. But I couldn't even stand up. I needed to rest, so I folded my arms on the desk and put my head down onto them.

And wept.

When my study mate – a lovely girl called Ai – came into the room and found me in tears, she was aghast. She rushed to my side, slopping her mug of tea in the process.

'What's wrong?' she said, no doubt wondering who it was that had died.

'I'm having a breakdown or something,' I replied, because all seventeen-year-old girls are entitled to a bit of melodrama. To be fair, it did feel like my world was ending. Or at least, my world as I knew it. This wasn't a blip. This was my immune system telling my brain that it couldn't continue. I had to stop, Cambridge or no Cambridge. I had pushed my body to breaking point; now it was pushing back.

I phoned Mum. 'I have to leave school,' I said.

'OK,' she replied. 'I've just got one more patient to see, then my clinic's over. I'll collect you afterwards.'

'No,' I said. 'You don't understand. I mean, I have to leave school forever.'

*

Maybe 'forever' was putting it a bit strongly, but I certainly needed to take off the rest of the academic year. My A level exams were due to begin in six weeks, and there was no way I'd be able to sit them. I would have to drop out and start the year again in September.

A few days later, I was lying in bed, my bedside table littered with discarded A level revision notes and empty Strepsil packets, when my mum tried to placate me.

'A couple of months' rest and you'll be a new person,' she said. 'Just think how much older and wiser you'll be than the others.'

I stared at her. 'Others?'

'The year below,' she clarified. 'The pupils you'll be joining.'

She had said it to make me feel better, but it had the opposite effect. Up until that point, I had been thinking about nothing except recovering and trying to get to Cambridge. The fact that I'd be doing it with a whole new set of classmates hadn't occurred to me.

I started panicking. It wasn't that there was anything wrong with the year below; it was just that I didn't know them. More importantly, they would have a completely false impression of me. Even though many people in my current year had drifted away from me, they at least remembered the pre-illness, 'normal' Lily. By contrast, my new classmates would know me only as the pale, swotty freak who drifted through the school like a resident phantom.

What was I going to do?

Keep fighting, that's what. I would rest and get better. Then, when I returned to school in September, I would be glowing with such health I would dazzle them all.

The angel on my right shoulder was quick to accept my vision, but the devil on my left took more convincing. *They're already in their cliques*, it said. *And you're hardly Claudia*

Winkleman charismatic. There's no way they'll accept you. Then, from the other shoulder, *I'm sure they'll be a friendly bunch and anyway, you are perfectly capable of making new friends.*

As I wrestled with my thoughts, the afternoon turned into evening, then the evening into night. My parents had gone to bed ages ago. The house was dark and still. I pulled the bedcovers around me and tried to go to sleep. Then outside in the garden, I heard the yelp of a badger, so I got up and pulled back the curtain. All I could see was darkness. What time was it? I stretched over to my bedside table and switched on my lamp.

It was four o'clock in the morning! I'd been lying awake for hours. Why couldn't I drop off? *Listen, Lily, everything's going to be fine. Just go to sleep and get better.* I repeated this over and over, as if saying it enough times would make me believe it.

I prayed for calm, but nothing happened. So, I dug out my rosary beads. To be honest, they hadn't made many outings since my First Holy Communion, but I was desperate here. I asked God for a sign that it would all work out. I told Him I was going to turn on the radio, and I begged Him to do something to reassure me.

The strangest thing happened. As I tuned into Metro FM, a song was just starting: 'No Woman No Cry' by Bob Marley. When he sang the chorus about how everything was going to be alright, I began to sob. I was half comforted but half freaked out too, because I hadn't expected God to be *quite* so direct in his reply.

Eventually, exhaustion set in, and I fell asleep on a damp pillow.

I had the whole summer to convalesce. I was still far from being well, but I was determined to put my time to good use. So, I decided to learn to drive. After all, sitting in a car for the odd half hour, how taxing could that be?

Very, as it turned out. Just fifteen minutes behind the wheel was enough to make both my glands and my face swell up. And I wasn't the only one returning home pale faced. There are learner drivers who crawl along and come to a halt several metres from the line at traffic lights. Then there are learners who lack only for a white helmet to be called the new Stig. I fell into the latter category – as my father discovered to his dismay when he took me out driving.

'You both look like ghosts!' said Mum one time as we arrived back home after a session.

'I need a lie-down,' I said as I staggered up to bed.

'I need a stiff drink,' said Dad as he staggered to the drinks cabinet.

My mum decided a bit of sun would put some colour in my cheeks, so the three of us jetted off to the Côte d'Azur. It was my first (and only) holiday alone with my parents. I spent my time eating baguettes, strolling through bustling markets and paddling in clear waters while hermit crabs scampered around my feet.

But it wasn't the holiday it could have been. It seemed as if no part of my body would be spared the effects of my illness. For example, I am not the type to burn easily in the sun, yet on that trip, even half an hour outside was enough to make my skin blister. I had developed photosensitivity. Also, I couldn't tolerate alcohol any more. One glass of wine and

I was gone. And if you are going to get plastered, in front of your parents is the last place to do it.

Back in England, I was no longer just pale, I was pale and peeling. It was August; my eighteenth birthday was looming, and my two best friends since childhood were away travelling the world. But I wasn't going to miss out on celebrating. So, when the day finally arrived, I gathered together what friends I had left and put on my glad rags. What could we do that my health would allow? I knew that if I hit the town hard, the town would hit back harder, so instead I planned a meal at a nice little Italian, followed by some drinks in a couple of bars.

It began well. My friends and I were huddled around a table in the Italian on Claypath, laughing and clinking wineglasses in the candlelight. When our pizzas arrived, I found myself inhaling the heady scents of basil, oregano and happiness. But halfway through the meal I started flagging. I remember thinking, *oh no, I've still got the pubs to come.* Which isn't exactly the party spirit, is it?

Later, in a bar, I spotted a group of boys I vaguely knew. They were the type that skived and drank and did goodness knows what in the mistaken belief it made them the new Kurt Cobain. When one of them saw me, he puffed out his cheeks.

At first, I didn't realise it was aimed at me. Then the same boy elbowed one of his mates, nodded towards me, and puffed out his cheeks again. They all looked at me and laughed. I couldn't believe it. They were making fun of my swollen, glandular fever face. I squirmed.

The thing is, I had looked dreadful for the last ten months, and my face had been huge. But before that night, I had thought I was improving. In the bar, my friends hadn't seen the boys' shenanigans. I turned to one for support and said, 'Am I looking really awful?'

She studied me, then replied, 'To be honest, you are a bit thin.'

Wow, it got worse. 'I meant my face.'

'Oh, because you're so pale?'

So much for support. Why not just say it? I looked like a Chupa Chup lolly.

The night dragged on. A couple of my friends were now chatting up two men on the other side of the bar. I couldn't have cramped their style more if I'd put on a woolly Christmas jumper and tap-danced over to them. I watched them flutter their eyelashes as Mr Smooth and Mr Slick bought them a round of cocktails. Both sides knew exactly what they were doing. I was not needed here. Part of me was relieved about that, because I felt so ill. Eventually, the girls came over and asked if they could go on to a club with their dates. They looked sheepish, but I didn't actually mind. I needed to go to bed.

'I think I might head home,' I said.

'Come with us,' they encouraged.

'No, really, I have to get back.'

And that was the end of my eighteenth. No one can say I don't know how to have a good time. I hailed a cab. A girl called Jess came with me and, as it was my birthday, we shared a giant cookie.

No, don't feel sorry for me. It had sprinkles and everything.

Chapter 3

As September came around, people assumed I must be fully better. No one *ever* has glandular fever for eleven months, do they? But when the term started, I found myself facing the same old struggle to get up and out each morning. By the time I arrived at school, I needed a lie-down. Luckily, I was able to have one, as the girls' schoolhouse was for boarders as well as day pupils, and there were spare beds going.

I had been made a prefect – or 'monitor' as we called them – and I was delighted to be given this role. But I didn't have the health to carry out my duties; I wasn't even managing to get to half my lessons. When the teachers saw this, it was agreed that I could come and go as I pleased. If I could attend a class, then I would. But if I needed to go home, then I was free to do so. I was even told to skip assembly each morning so I didn't have to climb the steps to chapel. These arrangements were introduced to make my life easier, and I feel blessed to have been at such a caring school.

But some of my fellow students didn't like the fact that I was treated differently. To be fair, if they had genuinely thought that I wasn't ill, it might have looked to them as if

I were being favoured. My immune problems were too alien for most teenagers to understand. Their concerns centred around their love lives, their exams… Few had ever needed to consider their health.

All the teachers were fantastic, apart from one who became so frustrated about me missing her lessons that she reported me to my housemistress. Halfway through my first term, I was called to the housemistress's office. She asked me how I was choosing which lessons to attend, and I explained that I was prioritising the topics I had missed the previous year. The teacher who had complained was teaching areas that I had already covered.

When my housemistress heard this, she confided in me that she herself had only just recovered from glandular fever – so she understood first-hand what I was going through.

I felt at home in the girls' schoolhouse, despite all that was happening. Among the many kind and easy-going pupils were my study mate, Isabelle – a savvy new girl – and a fabulous boarder called Caja. Then, across the road in one of the boys' houses, was my boyfriend, Freddie.

You're probably wondering how I managed to nab myself a boyfriend while I was floating in and out of school with a pale face of varying proportions. As it happened, I had known this guy pre-illness; he had once closed me in a music practice room to tell me he loved me. I'm ashamed to say I was a bit cross about that at the time – it had made me late for chemistry. Freddie ended up showing compassion and understanding like no other boy in the sixth form. I felt I had an ally, and I decided to ignore the fact that we were totally unsuited.

As for Caja – well, at first it appeared we had little in

common. She was a bubbly blonde who spent all her time in the music school, whereas I was a studious brunette who spent all my time in the labs. Then, near the start of my repeat year, I went to an introductory coffee morning for girls and their mothers. It was a chance for everyone to get to know each other away from the heavy male influences of the school. I left my mum's side to go and get a custard cream, and by the time I returned, she was deep in conversation with Caja's mother.

Caja was there, too. I had never spoken to her properly, so we stood together nibbling our biscuits and smiling self-consciously while our mothers talked as if they were long-lost friends. They were discussing chronic illnesses.

'Glandular fever?' said Caja's mum. 'Caja was so ill with that. She spent some time in hospital on a drip.'

My ears pricked up. A fellow glandular fever sufferer?

'She hasn't been right since junior school,' Caja's mum went on. 'She has ME, you see.'

Now I was *really* surprised. Caja looked so… normal. Though now that I thought about it, I couldn't ever recall having seen her play sports.

Mum shared my own story. As she spoke about how little I was able to do, I saw the same surprise in Caja's expression. Her smiles became more natural and we were soon chatting together. We might have had different interests, but we had the same outlook on life. Perhaps we had both learnt from our time being ill what was important and what wasn't. We made a connection that afternoon that has lasted decades.

Towards the end of my first term, I was called back into my housemistress's office. She started to speak, then hesitated. I wondered what was coming.

'Lily,' she said at last. 'Some of the other monitors came to see me today. They think you're not pulling your weight. I hear you've missed some of your stints on the rota?'

'I've missed *all* of my stints on the rota,' I said. 'But I always let them know in advance, and I explained to them how ill I've been.'

The housemistress looked at me with genuine compassion. 'I did too, but I'm not sure they understood. They seem to think we should have picked someone more…'

'Healthy?'

I sympathised with her. Both she and I knew I wasn't up for the part of monitor. I wanted to make things easier for her. 'You'd like me to step down as monitor?'

'Not step down, more… move aside. We'll take you off all duties and make another girl monitor too. Is that OK?'

'Of course.'

I had to admit, it was a relief physically. But the moment was bittersweet. Previously, the pupils who'd complained about me had been all smiles and sympathetic hugs when my illness interfered with my duties. Now I wondered if that had just been for show.

*

It wasn't right. I was following all the medical advice, but a year after being diagnosed, I was still no closer to beating the virus. Every day, Mum came home from work with the latest unhelpful advice from her hospital colleagues. They told her I was right to keep pushing myself. They told her that I might be developing ME/CFS, but that the glandular fever virus (Epstein-Barr Virus or EBV) would definitely not still be active in my system. Instead, it would have gone into a kind of hibernation called 'latency'.

My body knew otherwise. I tried to tell my mum that I still had all my glandular fever symptoms, and she did listen. But she listened to her medical friends more. What did I know? I was just a school kid.

Yet, I was the patient. I was the only one who knew how I felt.

One day, I resolved to make her see things from my point of view. I found her tidying a pile of newspapers in the lounge, and I asked her to sit with me on the sofa. While I gave her my speech, she didn't take her eyes off me. Then, when I finished, there was a moment of silence.

Eventually, Mum said, 'I know you feel ill. I know you think you still have glandular fever. But the virus goes dormant after several months. You're just struggling to get your energy back.'

'Are you talking to me as a doctor or as my mum?'

'Both.'

'Well, I need you to listen as my mum.' I took her hands in mine. 'I *do* still have glandular fever and we need to do something.'

'But, sweetheart—'

'Sometimes I think that I'm… not dying exactly but – I can't explain. I just know I'm not winning the fight.'

Mum put her doctor face on. 'OK. We'll go to the GP tomorrow and ask for a repeat glandular fever test.'

'He thinks I'm fatigued.'

'We'll insist on the test and then you'll – I mean we'll – see.'

But I had heard her slip, and I was devastated she believed her medical friends over me. I knew I was alone on this one.

*

No – bloody – way. How could this be the case? The results were in from my repeat glandular fever test, and they were negative. I was sitting beside my mother, opposite a GP who was showing off all he knew about ME/CFS. He puffed out his chest as he droned on about graded exercise programmes. But I wasn't tired; I was ill. And not *differently* ill, but *exactly-the-same-as-a-year-ago* ill.

By then I'd read about ME/CFS in various articles. To be labelled with the condition, you simply had to have experienced severe disabling fatigue that affected your physical and mental functioning for at least six months. How vague was that? Plus, why was I being labelled with a new illness when the original one still fitted my symptoms perfectly?

I waited for the GP to pause for breath and then jumped in.

'But I still have my blobby face,' I explained. 'Sometimes my eyes are so swollen I can't even open them.'

'You should see my wife in the mornings!'

'And the nausea. After meals, I have to sit outside and focus on breathing so I don't throw up.'

'A levels can be stressful,' the GP said. If my head had been in range, I'm sure he would have patted it.

This wasn't stress, though. I was confident about my A levels – far more confident, in fact, than I was about his diagnosis. And as for his patronising demeanour… I had to get out of there before I was tempted to give him a swollen eye of his own. To add insult to injury, he suggested I take a course of antidepressants. I declined through gritted teeth and left the room breathing fire.

As I got into the car, I managed to close the door on my coat and had to yank it free. 'I can't *believe* he suggested Prozac,' I said to my mum.

'Won't you consider it?'

'Judas!'

Her gaze held steady on mine. 'I know you're not depressed – I *am* a psychiatrist. But the latest trend is to treat ME with Prozac. It might rev you up.'

'Do I look like I need *revving up*?'

'Not at this precise moment, admittedly.' And she gave a half-smile that only made my anger burn hotter.

'What do I have to do to get through to you?' I was shouting now. 'I – still – have – glandular – fever.'

Mum reached across the handbrake and took my hand. 'No, you don't. That's what the results showed.'

'Then the results are wrong!'

We didn't speak on the journey home. Our differences were like a wall between us. When we parked in our driveway, I got out of the car and slammed the door. Then, as I marched towards the front door, Mum lowered her car window and called out, 'Lily, come back here!'

I stormed across. 'What?' Was Mum going to tell me she had finally seen sense? Or maybe apologise for not trusting my judgement?

Instead, what she said was, 'Do *not* slam the door of my MX-3.'

So, I opened the house door and slammed that instead.

I stomped up to my room and flung myself onto the bed. Later, Mum came up to make peace, but it felt like peace was something I would never find. Under my duvet, I was seething. I racked my brain for ways that I could prove I still had glandular fever. I would have to find out all about the blood test the doctor had done on me – what it looked for, what the rate of false negatives was. Was there a different test I could have? All the while, I could feel my health draining away. I began to tremble.

When my mum returned to check on me, she felt my forehead and frowned. 'You're burning up,' she said. 'Let me get the thermometer.'

My temperature was a lofty forty degrees and rising. As the night drew in, the world around me started to melt. Mum telephoned the doctor on call. When he arrived, I was hallucinating. A tarantula the size of a dinner plate was crawling across the duvet towards me, and I looked around for something to bash it with. The doctor's voice seemed to come from the other end of the house. I dimly remember him telling my mum that I might have meningitis, and that if I developed a rash she should call another doctor immediately. He gave me paracetamol for my fever, then left. But as I was so busy battling a giant arachnid, I'm afraid my other memories of that episode have faded into the fever haze.

A rash did eventually flare up across my torso. On the plus side, my temperature started to recede, taking my hallucinations with it. By the time the tarantula was gone, a different doctor was perched at my bedside. His gaze flitted across the spots on my body.

'I'd know that rash anywhere,' he said cheerfully. 'You have glandular fever.'

Mum's expression harboured a hundred reservations. 'It can't be. She did contract glandular fever about a year ago. But she had a repeat blood test just this week, and it came back negative.'

'You mean the Monospot test?' The doctor waved a dismissive hand. 'Oh, I wouldn't pay any attention to that. No, Lily's rash is indicative of glandular fever, and if she has had it for a full year then she should be referred to an immunologist as soon as possible.'

Honestly, I could have snogged him.

*

Now that my mum believed me, she put out feelers to find the best immunologist in the area. She learnt that the da Vinci of the field was Dr Gavin Spickett, based in Newcastle. So, Mum arranged a referral, and within a week I was sitting in his waiting room, all blobby-faced and naïve. So naïve, in fact, that I even wore my school uniform in case he was about to lay his healing hands on me and send me to class afterwards.

My first impression of Dr Spickett was that he loved medicine as much as my mum did. It would be an exaggeration to say he was jumping up and down and clapping his hands together with excitement, yet his enthusiasm left a lasting impression on my eighteen-year-old brain. And he *listened*. So few doctors did that. I felt like I was in safe hands at last.

He explained to me that the routine blood tests for glandular fever (the Monospot/Paul Bunnell tests) weren't particularly sensitive. For my fellow geeks out there, I've gone into further detail in a footnote.[1] Suffice to say, when Dr

---

[1] The body responds to EBV by producing both specific antibodies to EBV *and* generic antibodies, called heterophile antibodies. The glandular fever blood tests that surgeries normally use (the Monospot/Paul Bunnell tests) detect the presence of heterophile antibodies. They can therefore throw up false positives (because heterophile antibodies are also produced in some other illnesses) and

Spickett arranged more specialised tests, they proved that, one year on, I was still in the acute phase of glandular fever.

It was wonderful seeing the proof in writing. I felt like pinning the results to the school notice board. I still had glandular fever! *Hurrah!* Now I could just swallow some pills, and the whole ordeal would be over before the time came to take my A levels.

It didn't occur to me to ask *why* I was still in the acute stages of the illness after twelve months. Nor did I wonder what sort of physical damage the virus might have done during its year-long rampage. Instead, I gratefully accepted from Dr Spickett my prescription for an antiviral drug called Aciclovir. It doesn't kill EBV – no medication does. But it slows down its replication so my body's immune system would have a chance to fight it. I had to take the maximum dose of the drug five times a day, dissolved in water. And I had to drink lots of extra water too, so that I didn't develop kidney stones from the medication. But finally, I was heading in the right direction.

*

---

false negatives (because they have to be carried out within a relatively small time window – ideally two to six weeks after contracting glandular fever). Moreover, some people with the virus don't produce detectable levels of heterophile antibodies anyway and have what's called heterophile-negative Infectious Mononucleosis. (Infectious Mononucleosis or 'IM' is just the medical name for glandular fever.) It is better to test for the EBV-specific antibodies e.g. the VCA antibodies. VCA IgM is produced in cases of acute infection and should disappear within six months. VCA IgG is produced at a later stage and stays in the person for life, so it is a good indicator of past EBV infection. Doctors sometimes look for early antigen (EA) and EBV nuclear antigen (EBNA) antibodies too, as these also help to show what stage the illness is at. When my results came back, they were positive for VCA IgM antibodies, but negative for VCA IgG. I was also positive for EA antibodies and negative for the EBNA ones. This showed I was in the acute stages of glandular fever.

Back at school, it was time for my mock A levels. I was determined to sit them because I wanted to see if my body could survive the rigours of a three-hour paper. Each day of the exams, I laboured up the steps to the exam hall with a bottle of water and a packet of Aciclovir. My tablets were so stubborn to dissolve, I had to stab the things with a teaspoon to break them up. Whenever Caja, sitting the exams with me, heard the tinkle of a spoon on glass, she would look around, and I would smile and signal for her to turn back so she didn't get into trouble.

After each exam, my health would deteriorate. But I knew the Aciclovir was working because, little by little, my face became thinner and my glands became smaller. When the exams were over, it was agreed that I should take a break from school so I could fight the virus properly. One evening, I rang my boyfriend Freddie to let him know that I would be back in school soon, and I asked what the gossip of the day was.

'You,' he said.

Oh no. 'What now?'

'You got ninety-eight per cent for your biology mock. I don't know whether to feel proud or ashamed. And you got a hundred per cent for one of your maths papers.'

I was as shocked as I was delighted. Had I shown the virus who was boss or what? But then I realised how the other kids at school would react. 'So, what is everyone saying?' I asked. 'That I'm not really ill? That I've been taking time out cramming and stuff?'

'Dunno. I've not been able to hear. Too busy getting ribbed for going out with a geek.'

That evening, I lay on my bed thinking it all through.

In the end, I decided I didn't care what people were saying. I realised that if I could get A grades when I was so ill, then going to the University of Cambridge was still within my grasp. All I had to do was continue taking my pills and keep it together when the real exams came. Then I could leave all this behind and start my new life.

At my next hospital appointment, my temperature was normal and my glands were nearly fully down. Dr Spickett suggested reducing my high dose of Aciclovir to a lower, maintenance dose, with the hope of later coming off it altogether. But when I tried doing so, my glandular fever immediately flared up again, so I settled back into my routine of five pills a day. I became so obsessed about not missing a dose, I wrote reminders to myself and left them scattered about the house. My brain fog couldn't hide them *all* from me.

It would be wrong to think of the pills as a silver bullet, though. At best, they were my bridge to the real world. My eyes remained sore, and my head still felt like it was filled with cotton wool. With my A levels fast approaching, I tried my best to revise. But now, everything I wrote seemed to bypass my brain. One morning, when I was feeling brighter, I dictated some A level notes onto a tape so that I could listen to it on the days when my eyes wouldn't open. Unfortunately, the sound of my voice droning on about bird-flight mechanics ended up sending me to sleep – as I suspect it would do to a lot of people.

As the summer term continued, I finally felt well enough to reduce my Aciclovir intake to the maintenance dose. But when exam time came around, I suddenly lost my self-confidence because there were several topics I hadn't yet managed to revise. On the day of my first A level paper, I drove to school and barged into Caja's room. I was holding an inch of notes between my thumb and forefinger.

'See these?' I screeched. 'I haven't even *looked* at them!'

Caja was lying on her bed, sipping Ribena while flicking through the latest *Cosmopolitan* magazine. 'See these?' she mimicked, holding up two whole lever-arch files. 'I haven't even *looked* at them!'

She always helped me keep things in perspective.

*

I remember very little about my A level papers. I don't know if that's because I was suffering from brain fog, or because they were not as traumatic as my health problems. But I did make it through every three-hour exam despite my glandular fever slowly worsening.

Now that work was over, it was time to have fun. At the end of the school year, each boarding house had a barbecue for its staff and pupils. It was now several weeks since my exams, and I was sufficiently rested that I felt able to go. I recall sitting on a picnic rug in the housemistress's garden, shouting to Caja over the reggae music blaring from a ghetto blaster, when we heard cheers from the boarding house across the road. The pupils there seemed to be having a much better time than us, so a few of the girls put their heads together and tried to think of some games we could play.

I can only assume everyone was high on Coca-Cola because, bizarrely, the game they decided on was… a cushion fight. The garden was littered with huge cushions for everyone to sit on, and soon people were being pitted against each other. The first one to knock down their opponent was the winner. Strangely, I was pitted against the teacher who had reported me for missing lessons. Perhaps whoever chose the match was hoping to create a little drama, but the contest worked wonderfully to clear the air between us.

When the games and food were finished, Caja and I found a quiet spot in the corner of the garden. We sat down on a wooden bench, in the shade of a tree, and Caja called a toast. 'To getting through A levels despite the illness!' she said.

'Cheers to that!' I agreed, clinking glasses.

And then we started to cry. The realisation hit us that we had actually made it to the end of school. All the lessons we had dragged ourselves in for, the throat pastilles we had sucked, the essays we had failed to complete… We had crossed the finishing line.

A couple of girls rolled their eyes, but we didn't care. What did they know about fighting a long-term illness? We wore our mascara tracks with pride.

When A level results time came around, my parents drove me to school. As I walked across the courtyard, I spotted classmates clustered around the tree outside the labs. Josh the maths whizz was bouncing around like Tigger, whilst Sam from biology class was inventing excuses for not going in. I made my way to the corridor where the results were pinned and scanned the lists for my name. My stomach was churning, and for once I couldn't blame my nausea on the glandular fever.

But the panic soon turned into relief. I had got the A grades I needed! *I was going to Cambridge!*

The next day, the local paper came to interview me. They

took a photo of me waving my A level results in the air. In the days that followed the story's publication, everyone gushed and said how well I looked. All I could see, though, was my facial oedema, which signalled that the EBV must still be active at low level. The paper ran an article on how I'd fought this dreadful illness and come out on top. It seemed a little premature to be writing the EBV's obituary, but everyone loves a happy ending.

I spent my last few weeks before university weaning myself off my Aciclovir crutch and coming to terms with all that had happened. In addition to my glandular fever ordeal, three other bad events took place over the summer: my house was burgled, my bearded collie died, and Freddie dumped me… via a mutual friend. I used to drive myself to Wharton Park – a historic park with views across Durham City – and sit by myself in the spot where all the bridal parties have their photos taken. I felt alone among the dog walkers, but I needed that fresh air and space to sort myself out. I could hear happy shrieks coming from the children's playground behind me. They reminded me of a carefree life, pre-illness.

Then one evening as I stared at the cathedral in the gloom, I started seeing my experiences in a new light. OK, so maybe I wasn't *totally* better. But I had been well enough to get the grades I needed, and I was well enough to leave home. In the future, when I was a successful researcher and, you know, polishing my Nobel Prize medallion, all this heartache would be forgotten. It was wrong for me to spend so much time dwelling on… what? An illness that had lasted less than two years? A failed relationship?

It was all over now.

So, I got back in the car and cranked the volume up on

the radio. As I drove home, I thought happily of Trinity Hall, of Darwin and DNA, and striding along King's Parade in the sunshine. No illness or boyfriend was going to sidetrack me.

Watch out, world.

Chapter 4

On a sunny October afternoon in '96, I was one of the first students to arrive at Trinity Hall for the start of Michaelmas term. After hugging my parents goodbye, I unpacked my bags and went for a walk around the college.

Trinity Hall is such a picturesque place, with tranquil courtyards and an immaculate lawn stretching towards the river. I looked at the college buildings, so orderly with their red-brick walls and their lead-paned windows. Parts of the exterior were covered with climbing plants, trimmed to complement the lines of the lawn. The only sounds were the calls of birds and the scuff of footsteps as students walked along the paths. I strolled down to the riverbank and stood among the trees, watching the punts on the River Cam drift by.

It was great being among students who were as geeky as me. Back at school, you were considered a swot for always handing your homework in on time. Whereas here, when the girl in the room next to mine saw my pile of Dawkins books, instead of teasing me, she asked to borrow one. On my first night, as I burrowed into the bed in my chilly stone room, I thought of all the students who had lain here before me and wondered if they had felt the same sense of belonging.

Then, like a gun firing, the term began, and I found myself rushing from lecture to tutorial to practical. On most days, I had morning lectures at nine, ten, and eleven, followed by a five-hour practical at the laboratories. Then it was back to college for write-ups, a tutorial, and an essay-writing shift before bed. It was an intense, yet magical time. I got on well with my tutors and the students both in college and on my course.

Sometimes, after an exhausting day's work, I would find myself having a meaningful chat with a boy in the darkness of someone else's room. Or as I was heading back from student night at the local club, I would at times forget my personal pledge to keep my distance from the opposite sex. And occasionally, just occasionally, I would accidentally kiss someone. But the next morning, as I closed the heavy wooden door of my staircase on the way to lectures, I would make a mental note to end any relationship before it began. I hadn't come to Cambridge to get a bloke.

I loved picking up the crisp sets of notes in lectures and personalising them with diagrams and annotations. I loved hearing the screech of stools as students rushed to take their places at the start of practicals. I even loved the smell of the enormous laboratories – the mustiness and the stench of chemicals that had built up from hundreds of years of experiments. I remember the first time I extracted DNA from cells by myself, spooling the long threads onto a glass rod. I felt like I was discovering life, and I imagined myself sitting in the same spot that Watson or Crick had occupied when they discovered the structure of DNA.

Then the physics students told me that that breakthrough had been made in the Old Cavendish Laboratory over on the New Museums Site – on *their* patch, in other words.

Gutted.

Not to worry, though. Maybe one day I would make my own discoveries, and people would think, *I wonder if this is where Lily sat when she discovered…*

I hadn't decided exactly what I would be working on, of course. I had to leave myself *some* surprises.

When I look back now, I wonder where the EBV was skulking all this time. I knew I wasn't well. Sometimes I had a swollen face or I felt disorientated, but it didn't stop me from going dancing or exploring Cambridge. Then again, I wasn't strong enough to join the university's ski club as I had planned, so I guess the best I could say was that I *nearly* had the EBV under control.

But would 'nearly' be enough?

*

'What are you doing tonight?' asked my friend Will as we waited for our quantitative biology lecture to start. Will was someone from Clare College next door whom I'd befriended – along with another boy, Bradley – during a fire drill at the chemistry department.

'There's a seventies night at Trinity Hall,' I said. 'I'm supposed to be buying some flares or a big-hair wig. So, if you have a way to get me out of it, please tell.'

'Do you like jungle music? There's a gig at Queen's tonight followed by a staircase party at Clare. But if you prefer ABBA—'

'I'll come with you,' I cut in. I had no idea what jungle music was, but I was looking forward to finding out.

'Great! We'll pick you up at eight.'

That night, I strode out of college in an insufficiency of clothing, grateful that my mum wasn't there to make me go back for my coat. Will and Bradley were waiting for me, and we walked to Queen's together through the backstreets of Cambridge.

'Aren't your legs cold in that miniskirt?' Will asked.

'I'm wearing opaque tights.'

'And obviously a thin layer of nylon is perfect insulation against the winter cold. They'll be wearing those tights on arctic expeditions soon.'

I covered a smile. 'You're supposed to be leching, not lecturing.'

He laughed. 'Just saying. Would you like to borrow my coat?'

'No. But thank you.'

Cambridge boys seemed so sweet.

We arrived early at Queen's. The dance hall was devoid of people, and lights flashed and bounced off the polished wooden floor. Earlier, when Will had mentioned jungle music, I'd pictured bongo drums and Tarzan yodelling. Instead, the tune that was playing sounded like someone had gone nuts in a drum factory. I went with Will and Bradley to the bar, and we caught up on science department gossip, then told dodgy jokes until my intercostals ached from laughing. By the time we returned to the dance hall, it was heaving.

Will dragged us onto the dance floor, where I learnt just how difficult it was to dance to jungle music with only two legs. I was smiling and swaying and—

Oh my gosh.

There he was: the loveliest guy ever. He had deep-set blue eyes and sculpted cheekbones, and he was dancing in a way that was both cool and self-conscious. He was a stranger, yet I felt like I knew him…

Oh no, he's looking! Act cool, act cool.

So, I averted my gaze and continued dancing.

But I soon glanced back. I couldn't help myself. Mystery Man was looking in my direction. I looked away again – just for a second, though even that took resolve. Then I looked back and—

No way, was he staring at *me*?

I danced with Will and Bradley, doing my best to appear casual. Yet when I glanced over at Mystery Man again, he was still looking at me. For a second our gazes locked. Then I remembered I didn't want a boyfriend. There just wasn't time in my life for a relationship. Maybe that would change after I graduated, but right now it would be unfair to lead this guy on.

Though when I *was* ready for a relationship, I would want to meet a man exactly like this—

'Earth to Lily,' said Bradley. 'Hello? We're going to the loo. Back in a minute.'

Apparently, it isn't just girls who go to the toilets in pairs. 'You can't leave me alone on the dance floor!' I shrieked.

'Then go and sit down somewhere,' said Will.

And with that my friends left me stranded.

A second alone on a dance floor feels like a lifetime, so I hurriedly scanned the room to see where people were sitting. Of course, the seating area was on the other side of Mystery Man. If I was going to reach it, I would have to walk straight past him.

Oh well, here goes…

As I passed him, I experienced a pull the like of which I'd

never felt before. And, geek as I am, I wondered if pheromones were to blame for me wanting to grab him and—

Stop it! Nice girls didn't behave this way. So, I carried on walking.

After I sat down on the floor, I tugged my miniskirt as far over my thighs as it would go to make myself seem less available. When I next looked up, Mystery Man was smiling at me, so I smiled back. Out of politeness, you understand. Then suddenly, he left his friends and walked towards me. He took my hand and pulled me up so I was face to face with him. I suppose I *could* have protested and made my escape, but next thing I knew, I was being led onto the dance floor. I didn't have to worry about my jungle-music-dancing technique because pretty soon we were kissing. I'm not sure that's the way Catholic girls are meant to behave, never mind girls who don't want boyfriends. But hey-ho.

You can imagine Will's and Bradley's surprise when they came back from the toilets. They had left me alone for only a few minutes, yet now I was absorbed with this stranger. I learnt that he wasn't a Cambridge student, and he learnt that I was Lily from Trinity Hall – though he kept calling it Trinity College and I kept having to correct him.

'Trinity *Hall*. It came *before* Trinity College.'

After hearing this for the third time, he arched an eyebrow, and it struck me that my chat-up lines might need some fine-tuning. But what the heck, something was working.

Eventually Bradley came over and tapped me on the shoulder. He said that he and Will were off to the staircase party, and that they would see me at lectures on Monday.

'No, don't leave me!' I hissed back. Look at the trouble that had got me into first time.

'You seem to be getting on fine without us.'

I felt tugged in two directions. I didn't want to risk the dark side streets on my own later, and I definitely wasn't going to invite a man – a total stranger – back to my room. But my friends made it clear that they were leaving, so I kissed Mystery Man goodbye, and I tried not to think about how I might be letting Mr Right slip away.

'What was his name?' enquired Bradley as we walked back to Clare College.

'Damn,' I said. 'I knew I'd forgotten to ask him something.'

The boys laughed, and I did feel foolish that my brain hadn't kicked into gear enough to ask something so obvious. It was the first time in my life that my heart had completely overridden my head.

When I woke up the next morning, I couldn't stop smiling at the memories from the previous night. Then I remembered I didn't know who Mystery Man was, or where he was from. Odds were, I would never see him again, so I might as well get on with writing my essay for that evening's tutorial. I had a shower, pulled on some clothes, then sat cross-legged in my armchair with my pen and pad at the ready. *Right, here goes.* Anaerobic respiration in C4 plants…

Oh, but he was perfect.

Over time, plants have evolved various mechanisms to overcome the harsh environmental conditions that nature subjects them to…

Is it really possible to feel this way? Now I can see why other girls make such a hoo-ha about their love lives.

C4 plants – that is, plants which use C4 carbon fixation – have a competitive advantage in environments that are arid or…

Sod this.

I wasn't going to be able to concentrate until I got this man out of my system. So, I grabbed another piece of paper and wrote a letter to Caja, describing what had happened at Queen's. Then I pulled on my coat (my mum would have been proud) and braved the chill November air to post it in the marketplace. I told myself that this was closure. I told myself that I needed to put this guy behind me, because I had work to do.

It took more willpower than I could have imagined. I had to turn off the love songs on Heart FM, even hang up my miniskirt out of sight in the wardrobe so it wouldn't remind me of him.

But the essay got written. I didn't drop my standards just for a bloke, you know.

*

In Cambridge, I didn't get much time to myself to think. Occasionally, I would wander down to the river and mull over everything that had happened in the previous two years. Compared with most of the other students, I had probably been through a lot. I had battled with my health, I had become aware of my mortality, and finally I felt free. Older. More spiritual, perhaps.

I had been brought up a Catholic, but I hadn't really thought about religion until I fell ill. I used to think that being spiritual meant going to Mass every Sunday. When I was young, my grandma would tell me that if I was really good, one day I might see a vision of the Virgin Mary or some other holy figure. I was so freaked out by the idea that

I vowed always to retain a naughty streak (while at the same time staying virtuous enough to remain on Santa's good list – it was a fine line to tread).

I considered becoming a member of Fisher House – the Catholic Chaplaincy for the University of Cambridge. I went along to their chapel and was warmly welcomed by a nun. She told me the group met frequently for lunch and chats, then showed me photos of some of their events. Her kindness and enthusiasm were obvious, but this wasn't my idea of faith. I needed space to think and pray, and I liked my social life to be filled with people who didn't all share the same beliefs that I had. So, I made my excuses and fled.

Instead, every Sunday, I made the trek to a different church on the other side of town – Our Lady and The English Martyrs – where people sang and shook hands but otherwise ignored me. Just the way I liked it (though, ironically, I did end up joining Fisher House subsequently when the hike across Cambridge became too much).

Once after church, back in my room, I pulled out my big grey notebook in readiness for writing up my most recent cellular biology experiment. I remember flipping through the pages of the book, taking in all we had covered that term. The first time we were handed back an assignment, the boy sitting next to me had punched the air and said, 'Ha!' He was desperate for me to ask him what mark he'd got, so naturally I made a point of staying silent. Instead, I looked at my own write-up. I assumed the tutor must have forgotten to mark it, because I couldn't see any red ink. Instead, all I saw was a strange symbol at the end.

It was… a fish. A little red fish.

Or was it a cross? My breath felt tight in my chest. Was

my work so poor that instead of wasting ink on it, my tutor had decided simply to put a cross on the last page?

Next to me, the boy had resorted to shoving his notebook under my nose in an effort to catch my attention. Clearly, I wasn't going to get any peace until I relented, so I said, 'What?'

'I got a beta!' he crowed.

And then the penny dropped: the lack of ink on my assignment, the symbol at the bottom – it wasn't a fish or a cross, it was an alpha. My mouth fell open, and I did a passing imitation of the fish I had mistaken it for.

I never told the boy beside me, of course. Pride can be a fragile thing, and I didn't want him sulking for the next five hours we would be sitting together.

*

As much as I enjoyed the mad rush of Monday-to-Saturday lectures, the undoubted highlight of my week was socialising on Saturday nights. One time, I had made plans to go to Henry's Café Bar for cocktails before returning to Trinity Hall for the weekly disco (we called them 'bops'). Things got complicated when Caja's boyfriend, Paul (who was studying at Cambridge too, albeit at a different college), approached me in chemistry lectures. He and a couple of his friends wanted to go to the disco, but they couldn't get tickets. Would I help them get in?

Unfortunately, I couldn't. I was only allowed to admit one non-college member – and then only if he went as my partner.

'I can't take all three of you,' I said. 'Sorry.'

But then Paul looked at me with his puppy-dog eyes, so I hatched a plan to smuggle them all in. I would go past the porter with Paul on my arm, then repeat the act with each of Paul's friends, hoping the porter didn't notice that my partner kept changing.

It worked a treat. That night, I got all three boys in before leaving for Henry's Bar with my college friends. For two hours, we caught up on the week's news while downing increasingly dubious cocktails of Bailey's and things that Bailey's should never be mixed with. Then we skipped and giggled our way back to Trinity Hall.

I swayed into the common room. It was packed with students jumping about to The Jackson Five's 'ABC'. There were kissing couples scattered around and the usual loud crowd showing off on a makeshift podium. Then, when I turned towards the bar, some bloke obstructed my path. I looked up.

And stopped breathing.

Not literally, you understand. I'm still alive (though it doesn't feel like it sometimes). But I'm not good with surprises, even pleasant ones, and it took me a while to register that Mystery Man was smiling down at me.

But… what was he doing here? He wasn't a Cambridge student.

My heart didn't care, but my head needed an explanation. My cautious side wondered if he had lied about not being from Cambridge when we first met so he wouldn't have to see me again. But no, if that were the case, he wouldn't be smiling now, he would be squirming. My spiritual side wondered if we were destined to be together, and if God had brought him back to me. But that was probably just the cocktails talking.

The cocktails...

My thirst had grown to just-crawled-in-from-the-desert proportions. I needed some water, and I needed it now.

Mystery Man said, 'Do you want to dance?'

Men always want the physical stuff so soon.

I couldn't speak. Eventually I forced my lips open just to see what came out. It had to be better than merely staring at him like a lemon, right?

'You're not from Cambridge,' I said, slightly accusatorily.

In retrospect, it would have been better if I had just kept staring at him.

He looked startled. Then he gave a half-smile and said, 'No, I'm not,' before leaning in and whispering, 'Am I allowed to be here? Or would you prefer it if I left?'

I didn't know what to say. My thoughts flowed like mud. Who was this guy? Why was he here? More importantly, why did I feel so alive in his presence? The need for answers competed with my need for a drink.

'So,' he said, interrupting my thoughts. 'Dance?'

Oh no, it was my turn to say something again. I didn't want a repeat of what had happened when I'd spoken just now. But nor could I face the prospect of dancing yet. Maybe after I'd had some water I would be able to take stock.

So, I said, 'No, I need a drink,' and strode towards the bar.

I assumed Mystery Man was following me. But when I got to the bar and turned to ask him what he wanted to drink, I found to my horror that he wasn't there. No, no, no, I wasn't going to lose him a second time. Why hadn't he come with me? I racked my brain. What had I said exactly? What I'd *meant* to say was, 'I can't dance now, but I'd love to later, so why don't you come to the bar with me and we can have a drink and chat?' OK, that wasn't *quite* what I had actually said, but surely he'd got the gist from, 'No, I need a drink'?

I bought a bottle of mineral water and hurried onto the dance floor, hoping he was still there.

Please, please be here.

He was. He was with two other strangers, blokes around his age, managing to look cool while dancing to 'Super Trouper' – which is no mean feat. For a while, I watched him with his friends, and I realised I felt the same about him as I had done at Queen's.

Right, that's it. I was going to grab him before he vanished again.

I strode across the room and tapped him on the shoulder. When he swung around, he looked surprised to see me. I opened my mouth to speak. I didn't care what came out this time, because there was nothing I could say that could make things worse.

Or so I thought. Because what I ended up saying was, 'Didn't you see me standing there?' Again, slightly accusatorily.

He looked taken aback, then amused, so I dragged him away to a quieter part of the common room and made my feelings clear.

*

'Lily, stop right there!'

I was walking down Trinity Lane on my way back to college when I heard those words. I knew that voice – Caja's – and I was thrilled to hear it in Cambridge. It was the following weekend, and Caja had come to visit her boyfriend Paul. I swung around, grinned and hugged her. She told me she had dumped her bags in Paul's college room, then immediately come out to find me.

'I want the gossip,' she said. 'Because I hear you've been up to all sorts.'

'Like what?' I replied, all innocence.

Her reply came out in one big, excited rush. 'When I phoned Paul on Sunday to ask if he'd spoken to you at the Trinity Hall disco, he said, "No, she was with her boyfriend." Boyfriend? I thought. So, I told him, "Lily doesn't have a boyfriend." "Well, she was kissing *someone*," he said.'

I felt out of breath just listening to her. 'Shall we go and get a pizza?' I said. 'I'll tell you the whole story.'

We made our way to the Italian in the market square with the white stone walls and the gingham tablecloths. Neither of us could concentrate long enough to read the menu, because Caja was itching for news, and I was equally keen to divulge. So, when the waiter came, we just ordered margherita pizzas and lemonades.

'So why did he come back?' asked Caja.

I explained, blushing madly, that he hadn't been able to stop thinking about me. He was at Law College in London, but his best friend studied at Cambridge, so Jon – that was his name – asked him how he could get to see me again. He knew I was Lily from Trinity Hall, so his friend told him my college was having a dance and somehow got them both tickets.

Jon had spotted me when he arrived at the start of the evening but had hung back to make sure I didn't have a boyfriend. You can imagine his surprise when he saw me telling the porter that not just Paul but also two other boys were my boyfriend. Understandably, he had been reluctant to become boyfriend number four. But then he'd seen me leaving alone for Henry's Bar, and he'd figured out what I was up to. So, he waited in Trinity Hall for me to come back.

'Can I be bridesmaid?' Caja joked.

'He's not even officially my boyfriend yet!'

'Look me in the eye and tell me you don't want to marry him and have his babies.'

She waited for an answer, but – would you believe it? – just at that moment the waiter returned with our pizzas, and I focused all my attention on the blobs of mozzarella melting into herby tomato sauce.

Afterwards, Caja and I ambled back to Trinity Hall.

'So, when do I get to meet him?' asked Caja.

'Who?' I replied, feigning confusion.

'Who do you think? The man who unleashed Lily!'

I raised my voice in mock outrage. 'Unlea— Look, if you mean Jon, he's coming to Cambridge next weekend for the Snowball.' The Snowball is a major social event held annually in Selwyn College. Tickets often sell out within hours.

'I'm going to that with Paul!' said Caja.

'Great! Then you'll get to see him there.'

*

Jon came back that weekend, and he did briefly meet Caja. But he and I spent most of our time alone, talking. I didn't know that it was possible to feel so at ease with someone who wasn't a close family member. Jon wasn't like the other boys I had gone out with. He was inwardly confident, yet outwardly shy. He knew his mind, and he understood other people too, but he never expected anything of anyone. And he kept his heart buried deep.

In those early days, we would spend hours at a time lying on my college bed with its cheerless brown covers, chatting and listening to The Cranberries or R.E.M. At first, we were both battling our feelings. I don't think Jon had been looking for a relationship any more than I had. He told me he generally needed space from other people, but he always wanted more time with me. One Wednesday, he left law lectures in London and drove straight to Cambridge on a whim, just because he missed me.

I found I could open up to Jon in a way I never had with anyone else. During our conversations, I came to realise that my illness had affected me more than I had appreciated. I was still as determined to become a scientist – in fact, even more so, just to prove to the virus that I had won. But I was more sensitive now. All my feelings were intensified. I noticed other people's struggles and insecurities where I would have missed them before. I guess I needed to have experienced hard times myself before I could detect that others had been through them.

Jon was a great listener. He was gentle and soulful. And to his surprise, he started opening up about his own past and his own struggles too. Through those conversations, in the glow of the oil burner and scented candles that littered my student room, we fell in love.

Each weekend, Jon came to visit me, and he would be waiting for me when I got out of Saturday lectures. I used to wear a miniskirt under my lab coat and keep some tinted lip balm in my pencil case. As I walked across the science site to meet him, I would take off my lab coat, untie my hair, and apply my balm. The transformation was swift and dramatic, from geek to chic. I felt like Wonder Woman.

In my last tutorial of term, the tutor handed back our most recent assignments and told the group to have a nice Christmas. The four of us stuffed our books into our bags and put on our coats. The others rushed for the door and I was about to head out too when the tutor said, 'Lily, could I have a word, please?'

As I watched the other three students troop out, my thoughts were a whirr. I couldn't imagine what the tutor wanted to talk to me about. I was normally such a good girl, but the times being summoned to see the housemistress at school had left me feeling paranoid. Had someone complained about me?

The tutor frowned. 'You know the essay I just handed back? "Why Be Mammalian?".'

I nodded, wondering where this was going. Somewhere with a sharp drop on the other side, probably. Then again, the tutor's expression appeared more pensive than disapproving.

'I set that same essay every year,' he continued. 'Sometimes for a tutorial, sometimes as part of the end-of-year exam. Yours was one of the best I've ever read. I thought you should know that.'

I stared at him, aghast, elated.

He grinned, lowered his voice and said, 'Happy Christmas,' before nodding towards the door.

I walked down the corridor with my heart hammering. A cleaner was pushing an industrial floor cleaner across the lino. I smiled at her, then danced out into the black December evening, trying to process the tutor's words.

The science site was empty. Most of the students were

back at college, getting ready for their end-of-term parties. The lecturers had gone home. I walked along an alley and onto King's Parade, past the shops and bakeries playing Christmas carols. Just then, it started snowing. I pulled my scarf tighter about my neck and let the emotions flood through me. I felt euphoric, liberated – like my whole life was coming together perfectly. Was this my reward for surviving my illness? I had never felt so proud in my life.

But you know what they say about pride.

Chapter 5

Just when I thought my life in Cambridge couldn't improve further, I found out next term that our lecturers would be taking us on trips to the Darwin Museum, the Botanic Garden and the Scott Polar Research Institute. I nearly passed out with excitement; one girl actually did.

No, not really.

I still smile when I remember the first time I entered the Darwin Museum. Its glass cabinets were bursting with specimens that Darwin had sent back to Cambridge from his voyage on the *Beagle*. I'd learnt this stuff in school, and it was a significant part of my degree course. But now I was looking at some of the actual creatures he had found – beetles, fish and insects, all suspended in glass jars and labelled in *Darwin's own handwriting*!

'That isn't Darwin's handwriting,' clarified one of the tutors. 'Lots of people think it is, but it was actually his servant, Covington, who did the labelling.'

OK, so not Darwin's handwriting. But these were still samples that he collected! Right here in front of me! It was sensory overload for geeks.

The trip to the Botanic Garden was equally thrilling.

Forty acres of flowerbeds, lawns and wooded areas waiting to be explored. At every turn, I was hit by an explosion of colour and scent. The lecturer handed each of us a free-entry pass, explaining that, as students of the university, we could come and go as we pleased. I couldn't believe it. My degree course was a gift that kept on giving.

Sometimes, I used to walk all the way to the Botanic Garden to plan my assignments. Unfortunately, all this tramping around Cambridge was beginning to take a toll on my health. My eyelids and chin swelled up, and on the way back from the Botanic Garden one day I felt so unwell I had to sit down in the street. Reluctantly, I decided to stay closer to college in future. Looking back, I can see that my symptoms were caused by the EBV resurfacing, but the joy of studying science carried me through to the end of term.

In the Easter holidays, I decided to go on one of the university's field trips to Pembrokeshire. These outings were not compulsory, but they were strongly recommended, and who wouldn't want to go on a trip like that? Seven days on a rugged coast with like-minded friends collecting sea invertebrates... Heaven!

So, a week later I boarded the first of three trains that would take me to the Welsh coast. I spent most of the journey reading my Collins guide to the seashore and eating a cream egg while thinking how much bigger these things had been when I was a girl. On my final train, I spotted my friend Bradley from Clare College and staggered down the juddering carriage to plonk myself beside him. He greeted me with a smile, and we compared notes on how many Easter eggs we had eaten in the last week. Gradually, other Cambridge students came to sit with us. By the time we arrived at our destination we had morphed into one big gaggle.

The hostel where we were staying was in a stunning location on a craggy cliff top overlooking the beach. Growing up in Durham, I had seen my fair share of dramatic scenery – we have a beautiful coastline, rugged moorland and forests galore. Yet there was a wildness to this part of Pembrokeshire that was completely new to me. As I dismounted the minibus outside the hostel, I heard waves crashing against the cliffs and felt the wind whipping around me. It was a reminder that here the elements ruled.

After unpacking our bags, we were given a talk by one of our lecturers about what we would be doing in the coming week. In the mornings we would collect samples. Then in the afternoons we would relocate to a research centre near the hostel to identify and record our findings. It sounded simple enough. However, the trek down to the shore and then up, up, up again to the laboratory turned out to be an enormous struggle. I remember aches firing down my limbs as I walked across the sand dunes, then the feelings of depersonalisation as I perched over my microscope in the research centre.

But I remember more how I felt when I was down on that beach with the cold air stinging my nose and the sea water numbing my hands. As my lab partner and I laughed and shouted over the wind, I knew I'd found my utopia.

Every evening, I went down to the hostel's dining room with the other students for our main meal of the day. The banter, the smell of lasagne and greasy chips, every detail has stayed with me because I think this was the last time for many years that I felt complete. After dinner on the second day, my friends decided to take the path down the hill to the nearest village. They knew of a pub there where the locals played fiddles and sang folksongs. 'And,' one of the boys added, 'the wine is *really* cheap,' as if that would sway my decision.

He knew me well.

By now, though, I had a feverish chill and a raging throat. There was only one way this was heading, so I made my excuses and watched my friends disappear into the blackness. Once their voices had faded, I headed inside and went to bed.

The next morning when I woke up, I had a temperature and a football-head. I knew it was game over. The other girls trotted off for breakfast without me, and five minutes later there was a tentative knock at the door of my dormitory.

'Lily? Can I come in?'

It was Bradley. He had heard I was ill and had come to check up on me. He was the only one in the group who knew about my glandular fever history.

'Do you think it's a full relapse?' he said as he hovered beside my bed.

I nodded.

'Will you be alright?' he asked softly.

I shrugged – partly because it hurt my throat to talk, but primarily because I had no idea of the answer.

Bradley urged me to go home. He said he would inform the lecturers so I could get on with packing. The moment he left, I began sobbing. I knew it was my fault that I had fallen so far. I had ignored the signals my body was giving me so I could chase my ambitions. But was gunning for my dreams such a terrible thing? And wasn't that the way I had been advised to get better from my illness? By pushing myself?

A taxi took me to the local railway station, and I had to endure the interminable journey back to Durham alone. To cheer myself up, I pictured returning to Cambridge in full health for the summer term. I thought about how I could make that image a reality. I would have to go back on the Aciclovir, of course, so the first thing I did when I returned to Durham was arrange an appointment with my immunologist.

Even after all these years, I can still recall Dr Spickett's look of disbelief when I entered his office, pale and round faced. Normally, once his patients improved to the extent that I had, that was the end of their story – they were better. Whereas it seemed like I was trapped in a time loop. Dr Spickett scribbled out a prescription for Aciclovir and told me to start taking the pills immediately. Before I left his room, I tried to convince him that all I was experiencing was a blip, and that I would be back at college very soon.

My blood test results subsequently confirmed that I was back in the acute stage of glandular fever. Nevertheless, university was due to begin again in a couple of weeks, and I intended to be there.

*

Returning to Cambridge for the summer term, I decided to go cold turkey on the Darwin Museum and the Botanic Garden – one trip and I would have only wanted more. Now, even walking was a struggle, and sometimes I had to take a taxi just to get across town. My work wasn't suffering, but it was taking longer to complete. When Jon visited at weekends, he gave me space to write my assignments so I wasn't cramming on Sunday evenings.

Then one afternoon, as I was resting before a chemistry practical, I found I couldn't get off my bed. My body wasn't paralysed, but there was no strength left in my limbs. I grabbed my make-up compact from the bedside table and flicked it open to look in its mirror. My freckles stood out sharply against swollen, translucent skin. The EBV was back angrier than ever.

'You need vitamins!' said my friend from across the landing.

'And soup!' said the French girl next door.

'And caramel shortbread!' said a student from the next staircase who had come along later to see why I had missed my chemistry practical.

I accepted their offerings with gratitude in the hope that these consumables would be all I needed.

But neither vitamins, nor soup, nor – amazingly – caramel shortbread made any difference. The following day, I felt sick. I wanted to blame the shortbread, yet it could have been the EBV playing havoc with my liver again. As I lay shivering under my duvet, I admitted defeat: I had to go home. I told myself that if I got some proper rest in Durham, I would be able to return to Cambridge for the end-of-year exams. Then I could continue with my degree as normal.

With the help of friends, I arranged a leave of absence from college, and before I knew it, my dad was knocking on my door to take me home.

*

I didn't get better in time to sit my exams. It took a couple of months just for my fever to abate, and that was on the high-dose Aciclovir.

During this time, a lot of correspondence went back and forth between me, the university, and Dr Spickett. I was granted a pass into year two despite the fact I had missed the year-one exams, and I am grateful to my tutors for being so compassionate. Cambridge has a reputation for being challenging, and yes, it was a very intense environment. But the source of pressure was the complexity of the work, not the tutors. In a letter to me, my senior tutor wrote: 'It is important though to remember that you are more important than the exams.' I'm trying to work out why I am welling up as I read that. I think it's because I didn't appreciate the value of health at the time. I wish I had.

Once I knew I would be able to continue my studies next year, I relaxed. Now I had the whole summer to knock the EBV on the head.

I *did* start to recover from the glandular fever. But like a car just out of its warranty period, my body developed a set of increasingly bizarre faults. For example, whilst my temperature came down when I was on Aciclovir, instead of then levelling off, it continued to sink. To stop myself shivering, I spent each day hunched up beside a radiator in my parents' lounge. My brain fog returned, but it wasn't the usual depersonalised sort, it was a new twenty-points-off-my-IQ sort. My mind was unable to solve the simplest of problems, like the order of events needed to make toast. And I would often say the wrong word without noticing. I also put on weight at a time when my appetite was unnaturally low.

The consensus of every doctor I went to was that I had developed ME/CFS. At that time, this appeared to be nothing more than a catch-all label for people who were struggling to recover from a long-term illness. It annoyed me immensely that it was often used irrespective of a patient's symptoms. Impatient for a better diagnosis, I read my mum's clinical medicine book and stumbled on a section about Hashimoto's thyroiditis. Hashimoto's is an autoimmune disease caused by the body attacking its own thyroid gland. As autoimmune disorders sometimes develop after EBV infections, it seemed a plausible explanation for my symptoms, and a blood test subsequently confirmed the diagnosis. I was prescribed Thyroxine tablets and told that my condition would improve.

But with the start of the new academic year approaching, my levels of thyroid hormones remained low. Packing my bags took several days. I would fold a jumper, then need a lie-down; put the sandwich toaster in a box, then grab a nap. Once in Cambridge, my parents stayed to help me unpack. After finally saying goodbye to them, I closed my door and slumped into a chair.

Hypothyroidism messes with your brain chemistry so you lose control of your emotions. At that time, I found that I would cry at the slightest thing. Then five minutes later I would forget what had caused me to weep – so I would cry about that instead. I increasingly chose to be alone because I didn't have the energy to talk. Friends came to see me, but I couldn't always keep up with their conversations. Walking to lectures, I would watch the other students whizz past on their bikes while I struggled to put one foot in front of the other.

This metabolic fatigue I was experiencing was poles apart from my viral fatigue. It was like someone had removed my batteries. My senses had also been dialled down. In lectures, I had to sit at the front of the auditorium so I could hear the lecturer properly. But halfway through a scribbled sentence, I would lose my train of thought and forget what she had said anyway.

Three weeks into term, Jon came to visit and hardly recognised me. He encouraged me to go home. By this stage, my hypothyroidism must have extinguished all my fight, because I yielded with barely a whimper.

Before I knew it, I was back in Dr Spickett's office. I learnt that my level of thyroid hormones had dropped even lower, meaning I now needed a much higher dose of thyroxine. The following month was lost to a zombie fog. My mind was like sludge, and my hearing showed no signs of improving. During one of my phone calls to Jon, I remember him talking about his 'bad son'. In my confused state I panicked, thinking he had a child he hadn't told me about. Whereas, in reality, what he'd been talking about was his bad *thumb* – an injury he had acquired playing football.

Slowly, my levels of thyroid hormone improved, and my personality returned. I wanted to go back to Cambridge immediately, but my body had other ideas. The parts of me that hadn't already succumbed to glandular fever or hypothyroidism were now desperate to get in on the act. I endured stomach cramps almost daily. My joints became stiff and sore. Then one day some of my fingers turned white and I lost all feeling in them. The cause turned out to be a circulation problem called Raynaud's disease. But my stiff joints and stomach pains remained undiagnosed. My skin also became oversensitive. Whenever I leant over, I developed red lines across my torso as well as itchy spots (or hives) around the lines.

Every so often I would try to pack my bags for Cambridge, but I never made it past a pair of jeans. As the weeks went by, it became clear that I would not be able to return to university any time soon. It was decided I should take off the rest of the academic year to recover; I could restart my second year the following autumn. The prospect of skipping a year wasn't as daunting as it might have been because I had done that already at school. I was still devastated, of course. But I was also relieved that my college wanted to keep me on.

Jon visited me in Durham every other weekend. We talked about me returning to Cambridge, and those conversations sustained me through the bleakness. Once, when Jon asked about my plans after graduation, I explained that I wanted to do a PhD.

'But you don't have to do that in Cambridge, do you?' he asked.

I didn't *have* to, but that had always been my plan. I never wanted to leave Cambridge. Someday, I intended to be a researcher or a lecturer there myself. But as I was about to explain that to Jon, I noticed he was watching me closely. And I realised there was something in my life that mattered even more to me than staying in Cambridge.

'No,' I said. 'It doesn't have to be Cambridge. There are good universities in… other cities too.'

'Cities like London, for example?' he asked.

'Cities like London,' I agreed, with a grin.

So that was my new plan. After graduating from Cambridge (a year later than intended) I would do my PhD in London while living with my hotshot lawyer boyfriend.

Just so long as I knew. I'm not good with surprises, remember.

Chapter 6

After the personal freedom of living in Cambridge, moving back home came as a shock. It was the same for my parents. In the absence of me and my brother, they had rediscovered a social life. Mum claims never to have stopped worrying about me when I was in Cambridge, yet her busy working week and her stream of dinner parties seemed to have got her through. She looked radiant in her party dresses, especially since she had reached her target weight for the first time in years.

'How did you get so slim?' her friends asked her.

'I sent my sick daughter to Cambridge,' replied Mum.

It was all down to stress.

My parents thought they should cut down on their socialising now that I was back, but I was determined not to spoil their fun. Once, I literally had to push my mum out the door while she said things like, 'Ring us if you need us,' and, 'We're only five minutes away, aren't we, Ian?'

'Well, about fifteen minutes, actually,' replied Dad.

'Not at the speed you drive.'

'Just go!' I said, laughing as I shoved Mum's sequinned shawl into her hands.

Then I returned to the lounge, dimmed the lights, and watched MTV in my dressing gown.

It was like this weird role reversal from when I was younger; my parents would go out partying while I kept the home fires burning. Occasionally, they would stay out all evening, and I would hear them creeping in at eleven like a pair of drunken teenagers. But more often, they would find some excuse to come home early. I remember them once returning at half past eight when they had only left at seven.

'It wasn't very good,' said my dad as he loosened his tie and poured himself a whisky. 'We thought we'd have more fun at home with our daughter watching' – he glanced at the television – 'pop music? So, er, who's this, then?'

Naturally, Mum appeared at that moment to fulfil her role in the double act. 'Has Dad told you tonight wasn't that good?'

They probably thought I believed this ritual, but I understood the sacrifice they were making. I started to appreciate them in a way that I hadn't previously. They weren't just great parents, they were great people too.

Jon continued to come up to Durham every other weekend. Our reunions were like something out of a war movie. Jon would step off the train, ashen faced after a hard week in the City, and I would dash towards him, pale and blobby and exuberant. Usually, we would spend the weekends cuddled up together, chatting about life or watching films. But if I had a shred of health, Jon would drive us to the coast, or to the depths of Northumberland. Once, we ended up on Lindisfarne. There's an ethereal quality to the island that makes you forget the rest of the world.

I had planned to visit Jon as often as he visited me, but

my glandular fever was having none of it. Sometimes I drove to the train station to buy my ticket, only for the drive and the queuing to knock me back so much I couldn't travel. On the few times I *did* make it to King's Cross, I would stagger off the train and look for Jon's pinstriped suit among the crowd. When he spotted me, his metamorphosis was striking; his depressed face would light up and become so unbelievably handsome that I'd have to catch my breath.

As a Durham girl, I never felt at home amid the stress and pollution of London. So many people looked hassled or defensive. Jon was determined to show me the city's brighter side. So, one morning he ushered me onto the tube and told me he was taking me somewhere I'd like. When we emerged above ground, he pointed to a distant grey building with lines of children outside.

'No way!' I shrieked as we joined the hordes converging on the London Aquarium.

Inside, my inner geek took over. I stared at the brightly coloured fish in the tanks, completely mesmerised. Jon, by contrast, spent most of his time staring at me and smiling at my reaction.

'You're so cute,' he said.

'Don't you think they're amazing?' I replied, gesturing to some horseshoe crabs.

'I'd rather see them in their natural habitat. I've always wanted to go scuba diving. But you know how it is. College, work. Maybe one day.'

'One day you'll die. Or catch a virus that makes your dreams impossible.'

'And there I was thinking you were my ray of sunshine,' Jon said.

He probably forgot immediately about the conversation, but I had mentally clocked his words and resolved to do something about them. Because if there is one thing I have learnt from my illness, it's that you have to do the things you want while you can.

*

Being back home with my parents wasn't *all* bad. Aside from anything else, it meant I got to have more contact with my grandma, who always kept me smiling. Grandma lived in Dublin but was frequently on the phone to my mum. In an effort to heal me, she tried persuading me to take cod liver oil. Then she instructed me to look in the mirror every day and *tell* myself I was better. I gave it a go once to humour her, but the ghoul looking back at me laughed in my face.

Next, Grandma started sending me holy water and relics from her pilgrimages to Lourdes and Knock. Among them were various medallions on strings. I was grateful to her for thinking of me, of course. But they looked like something she had picked up at a flea market.

'You are wearing them, aren't you?' she asked me one day on the phone.

'Not exactly,' I replied. 'I've hung them on my wardrobe door.'

'Well, at least your clothes will be healed.'

I wish that Grandma were still here now. I would tell her that I am praying and taking my fish oil every day, and that I finally understand the need for holistic healing.

The strangest of Grandma's 'gifts' was yet to come. One

night, Mum called me into her room, and I trotted in and sat on her bed. She produced a transparent bag that Grandma had sent her with a piece of discoloured material inside.

'I need to place this on you,' she said.

'A dirty hanky?'

'Lily! It's at times like this that I think I should have sent you to a Catholic school.' Mum opened the bag and took out the cloth. 'This is a first-class relic of Padre Pio.' She pointed at some blotches. 'Look, this is his actual blood! Now come here and I'll put this on you.'

'No way!' I said, jumping off the bed. I didn't want to add a Staphylococcus infection to my list of problems.

Ignoring my objection, Mum leant towards me… and in doing so almost fell out of bed. We both giggled. Then Mum's expression turned serious.

'I dread to think how many strings Grandma pulled to get a relic as precious as this,' she said. 'But she did it for you because she wants you to get better. And she believes, as I do, that it might help.'

I sighed and put my hand on hers – on her hand that wasn't holding the relic, that is. I wasn't going anywhere near *that*. 'If God wanted to heal me, he wouldn't need a bit of material to do it.'

Mum wasn't backing down. 'I think,' she said, glancing at the cloth, 'that if an elderly lady goes to that much trouble to help you, the least you can do is try it.'

That's the trouble with having a psychiatrist for a mother: the mind games. I never stood a chance. So, I let her place the rag over the biggest glands in my neck, then made my getaway.

The following morning, I was woken by the creaking of

my bedroom door. A mop of blonde hair appeared around it.

'Sorry,' whispered my mum, ducking back and closing the door again.

What the…? My parents never disturbed my convalescing sleep. Normally, they crept around in the morning, though in reality my dad would forget the rule after ten minutes and start crashing about in the kitchen until Mum told him off. So why had she woken me today of all days?

Then I remembered our discussion the night before.

I forced myself out of bed and downstairs. Mum was sitting at the kitchen table, nursing a cup of coffee. I didn't need to tell her I wasn't cured. One look at my swollen eyelids told her all she needed to know.

'Did you honestly think it would work?' I asked.

'I'd hoped,' she replied. 'Don't you feel any better at all?'

At that moment I wanted to feel better more for her sake than for mine. 'No,' I said. 'Sorry.'

'Not even *slightly* less brain fogged?'

'No.'

'Oh,' said Mum, looking back at her coffee.

So, I put my arm around her and whispered, 'But it doesn't mean I won't *get* better.'

*

I did everything I could to do just that. I stayed positive. I rested on each of the twelve days between Jon's visits. I ate and slept well. But my health problems weren't resolved, especially my hypothyroidism. I wasn't quite the neurotic deaf lugs I had been before starting on thyroxine, yet my other symptoms were proving stubborn to shift.

One bleak day in December, I was huddled in bed when my mum came in.

'You're so pale,' she said, grabbing my wrist and checking my pulse. 'It's forty-four! How do you feel?'

'Dreadful.'

'This isn't right.'

A pulse of forty-four indicated my health had crashed to a whole new low. Within a week, I had got an appointment as an inpatient at the Royal Victoria Infirmary's Programmed Investigation Unit. I didn't want to go. I hated hospitals, with their stink of disinfectant and their aura of death. But a couple of days before Christmas, I found myself lying in a hospital bed with a needle in my arm. They injected me with various hormones, then collected blood at regular intervals to check my body was responding correctly. I also had a chest X-ray and a brain scan, along with a battery of other tests I have banished from memory.

It was one of the worst times of my life – and there has been some stiff competition on that score. It was Christmas. I was twenty years old. Yet there I was, stuck in hospital with the eighty-year-olds doing sudoku and the nurses passing around the Quality Street. My friends were out buying dresses for their Christmas parties. My boyfriend was in London, working in his swanky office with beautiful, intelligent, healthy people. I felt utterly alone, not to mention old before my time. I tried to draw the curtain around my bed so I could have a cry in private. But then a nurse came striding towards me. No doubt she'd remembered a part of my body she hadn't yet stabbed a needle into.

She was carrying a box. 'Parcel for you,' she said.

I thought she was joking. I half expected her to open the box and whip out ten empty vials for my blood.

But no, she left the parcel on my bed and departed.

I stared at the hospital address scrawled on the box's label. When I recognised Jon's handwriting, my spirits lifted. I knew that, out of everyone in the world, he would understand how I felt. Within moments, I was hacking at the tape around the parcel. Inside was a big, cuddly Winnie the Pooh (I had a soft spot for that fat bear), together with a cassette. I grabbed my Walkman, inserted the cassette, then pressed play. It was a compilation of songs that Jon knew I liked, and others he thought I would. That tape helped relieve the awfulness of the next twenty-four hours. But even more, the sentiment behind the gift made me realise that not everything in my life at that time was shades of black. Before I fell ill, science had been my driving force; now it was the love of those close to me that carried me through.

The next day, the results of my scans and blood tests began to trickle in. For the most part, they were normal. I'd read in medical journals that researchers had found small lesions (called UBOs) in the white matter of some ME/CFS patients' brains, and I didn't fancy any of those. So, I was delighted to hear my brain scan was normal. But by the time my final test results arrived, I started to feel a bit disappointed. I had endured two lonely days in hospital for… what? Was there to be no resolution?

'So, these tests proved nothing?' I asked the endocrinologist who had come to deliver the news. He was a slender man with rolled-up sleeves and a down-with-the-kids attitude. He pulled a chair over and sat down.

'Not *nothing*,' he said. 'They've shown that you've got polycystic ovarian syndrome, and that you're not converting enough of your Thyroxine into a form the body can use.'

I was eventually prescribed a different type of thyroid medication – Liothyronine – to take in addition to my usual Thyroxine pills. And I was referred to a gynaecologist about my ovaries. But something told me the crux of my illness had still been missed. We had vanquished mere henchmen while the 'big bad' remained at large.

*

My dad collected me from hospital and drove me back to more months in my sick house. Taking the new thyroid pills marked the start of my recovery from hypothyroidism. But virally, I was slipping further backwards. Then my health faced a new challenge from a most unexpected source: visitors.

There was a time when I thought I should take every phone call and welcome every person who came to my door with tea and Hobnobs. When I did so, though, I would invariably relapse afterwards – sometimes for a day, sometimes for weeks or more.

'Why don't people understand how much I need to rest?' I asked my mum.

'Have you told them?' she replied, which was fair enough. But even when I did, they still didn't get it. They would say things like, 'Don't worry, I haven't got long anyway,' then proceed to talk to me for fifty minutes. It was too much for my body to handle. Some visitors genuinely came to see how I was, and I was so grateful for their kindness. But others talked *at* me. Unlike their other friends who were at work or in lectures, I was always available whenever they wanted to vent.

Sometimes my friends wouldn't even ask how I was. Or they would make comments like, 'You're not *still* ill, are you? But it's been ages!'

Thank goodness I had people to remind me of that fact.

Occasionally they would twist the knife with, '*Nobody* is sick for that long.'

To spare myself such remarks, I would sometimes not discuss my health at all. At other times, I couldn't discuss it because I had already used up my day's health allowance sorting out their problems. And I never phoned any of my friends myself because I would always still be recovering from their last call. I got told off over and over for that. Apparently, I never shared my news with them. A close friend actually said to me, 'Do you know why I used to like you, Lily? Because you were fun. Now you're just boring.'

She isn't a close friend any more!

One of the last things she said to me was, 'Isn't it amazing how the people you think will go far in life turn out to be the ones who fail?'

I didn't have a clue what she meant. 'Sorry?'

'I had this friend who went to Oxford and got ill,' she said. 'Now she's stuck at home with her mum. She'll never get better either.'

Either. The word stung. I didn't like being written off when I'd only been ill for a couple of years. Mind you, I was both surprised and flattered to be included in this imaginary group of high achievers. You have to take the rough with the smooth.

I wanted to know more about this Oxford girl. 'What's wrong with her?' I asked.

'Dunno. Your sort of illness.'

I wondered if she existed at all. My friend had a history of bending the truth, and she seemed to take a perverse pleasure in my plight – as if knocking me down made her feel better about herself. On the other hand, if this Oxford girl *did* exist, how many people like me were out there, catching viruses and never regaining health?

Two people whose visits I truly appreciated, however, were my parish priests. They took it in turns to come and sit self-consciously in my dad's armchair, and the air of hope and calm about them was tangible. One time, though, the more loquacious priest let something slip that troubled me; he told me that my mum had been crying in church. For a while, I wondered what to do with this information. Eventually, I decided I had to talk to Mum about it.

'Oh, it's just me being silly,' she said. 'When I'm praying for you, it gets a bit emotional.' And she changed the conversation so abruptly that I had no choice but to leave it there.

But it left me with scars that were slow to heal. My mum was so reserved, the last person to cry in public. What was my illness doing to those around me?

It seemed that the people in my life fell into two groups: the ones who were living the illness with me and being gradually broken down by it, and the ones who didn't appreciate what I was going through. Despite my efforts, it became apparent that there was nothing I could do for either group. Friends from university who wanted to visit me got fed up waiting for me to recover. Others slipped away because I was too ill to reply to their letters or emails. Eventually, the only people I had left were the ones who stood by me no matter what – who were able to see the real Lily behind the swollen, white face.

As the months passed, my hypothyroidism continued to clear. I could hear properly again. My thyroid brain fog lifted sufficiently for me to speak coherently. Now I just had to get rid of the viral symptoms. I drew a big sketch of the Epstein-Barr Virus and stuck it on my wardrobe door with the word 'DIE!' on it. Sometimes I would snatch a thick black marker and stab it and scribble on it.

But the virus had the last laugh. By the following Easter I was back on the full dose of Aciclovir.

One day in May I was lying on my bed watching a bluebottle headbutt the window when the phone rang.

'Come away with me.'

It was Jon. Even his voice made me feel happier. 'I can't,' I said. 'I'm fighting a virus.'

'Fight it in Malta.'

'I'd love to. But I'm not well enough. I can't even dress.'

'You dress to go to your blood tests.'

'And I definitely can't pack.'

'Your parents can help you.'

Well, that was true. But I didn't feel up to going away. 'Why do you want to go to Malta anyway?' I asked.

'Because the Med's a lot nicer than the Thames for diving.'

I had organised a scuba diving course for Jon in London as his Christmas present. To pass the course he had to do an open-water dive, and he wanted to do it over there.

Jon added, 'The hotel with the dive school overlooks the sea. It also has a spa and some therapy rooms. You could convalesce while I dive.'

It sounded sublime. 'I'm seeing my immunologist this week. I'll ask him if he thinks I could make it.'

'If he says yes, will you come?'

'OK.'

I could sense Jon's elation all the way from London. It seemed premature, though. When I saw Dr Spickett, I was sure he would say no.

As it turned out, he thought a break would be a splendid idea. And before I knew it, my parents were passing down suitcases from the loft. I had mixed feelings about going to Malta. I felt weak and lightheaded. It hurt to extend my arms or bend my knees, and my bowels were constantly knotted in pain. But Jon needed me and wanted to be with me, just as I needed and wanted to be with him.

More than anything, though, I wanted to get better. Maybe Malta would help?

Chapter 7

So, I found myself sitting on a balcony, staring at the sun setting over the Mediterranean Sea. The room had a beautiful view of Malta's capital city, Valletta, across the bay. The dome of its basilica dominated the skyline, reminding me of God's presence. I looked down at the promenade below. Here and there you could see joggers running alongside the rocky beach. Jon had intended to go for a run on his arrival, but instead he had drifted off to sleep after trying out the bed. Too many late nights at the office.

The name of our resort, Sliema, means 'peace' or 'comfort', but it was yet to bring me either of those feelings. It was crazy. Here I was, on holiday with the man I adored. I should have felt blissful, but I didn't. I felt like I had a hole inside me because there was an unwelcome guest on this holiday: my illness. It followed me everywhere, robbing me of my serenity.

The next morning, Jon looked refreshed. He was sitting upright in bed, reading about his diving school.

'I'll be gone all morning,' he said. 'Will you be alright?'

I pretended to consider. 'Hmm, let me think. The hotel has three restaurants, four pools, and a spa. I think I'll cope.'

Later, when he closed the hotel room door behind him, I collapsed onto the bed. The journey to Malta had knocked me back, and it was time to undo the damage. I grabbed the hotel's information pack and scanned the treatments on offer in its therapy rooms. Half of them I had never even heard of. I was a scientist, and to me alternative medicine seemed like something from a Harry Potter book.

Eventually, I settled on reflexology because it sounded like a glorified foot massage. Nothing too weird about that, plus it might help me relax. Apparently, it would also free my energy flow and flush away my 'toxins', but I took these claims with a pinch of salt.

So, I phoned downstairs and booked a session for later that morning, then hit the balcony to soak up some sun.

*

'You has problem wi' neck, throat, your – how you say? – glans?'

The reflexologist startled me, his accurate diagnosis cutting through the whale music.

'How can you tell?' I asked.

'The feet, they tell all,' he said. 'The glan' in the neck, 'ere,' – he pointed to his thyroid – 'it not work right. You know?'

Yes, *I* knew. But how did he?

'And your... er... 'ere.' He flapped his hand over his liver area. 'Leeva! Your leeva has too much, er... It work too 'ard.'

Well, I had to admit I was impressed. EBV affects the liver, and the organ was probably a bit overworked processing my Aciclovir too. 'Yes, it's had a lot to do recently.'

He nodded sagely. 'All in feet,' he said. 'Ovaries too.'

This was uncanny. How was he detecting my every ailment?

'Ovaries?'

'Yes, problem in ovaries.'

So much for the therapy relaxing me; my mind was now buzzing with curiosity.

'Anywhere else?' I asked, hoping he wasn't about to diagnose a problem I knew nothing about.

'No. I most tell ovaries an' leeva an' this glan' 'ere.' He pointed to his thyroid gland again. 'But I heal all.'

If only he could.

*

I was still pondering this the next day when I went on an 'underwater safari' with Jon. This took place on a glass-bottomed boat with an 'observation keel' below the water that allowed passengers to see the fish. As I strolled on board, the Maltese boatman slapped my cheeks with his leathery palms.

'You need go out more!' he exclaimed in his thick Maltese accent. 'You white!' And he laughed, oblivious to the fact that no amount of sunshine could alleviate the pallor caused by my illness.

As the boat sailed out to sea, I watched the hotels along the waterfront recede. Jon put an arm around me and pointed out our balcony in the distance. But I was still brooding over the boatman's laughter and the reflexologist's diagnoses…

Stop! I told myself. *Can't you just enjoy this trip?*

Unfortunately, I couldn't. As we left the bay, the wind

whipped up and the boat started to sway. Not much – I daresay I was the only one to notice it. But I suffer from travel sickness, and it is always worse when the EBV is active. I found myself struggling not to retch.

Soon, the boatman announced that we would go down to the observation keel. Tourists clambered towards the steep metal steps that led below while I remained clinging to the rail.

'Are you waiting until it quietens down a bit?' asked Jon.

I nodded in reply, fearing that if I opened my mouth at that point it might not just be words that came out.

But when people started chattering about the octopus they had spotted below, Jon took my hand and tugged me towards the steps.

'Come on, we might get to see it if we're quick.'

I didn't get to see the octopus because my nausea wouldn't allow me to stay in that stuffy, enclosed, swaying capsule for long enough. I had to come back up for fresh air. I waited on deck, taking deep breaths to curb my sickness. Around me, holidaymakers were taking photos and eating Magnums. I realised that I was now a spectator in life, not a player.

When I wasn't feeling nauseous on that holiday, my health actually began to improve. By the end of the fortnight, my stomach cramps had disappeared and my joints were pain free. As I boarded the plane home, I discovered my aches had completely gone. I remember the moment clearly. The flight attendant handed me a newspaper with a headline about Geri Halliwell leaving the Spice Girls. In my seat, I started to read the article, and as I turned onto page two, I realised my arm made the manoeuvre without discomfort. Curious to see if the pain was genuinely gone, I extended my arm into the aisle, bent it, then waved it in a circle – and narrowly missed whacking a young boy running past.

Something had happened in Malta to relieve my pains. I just had to find out what it was.

*

The day after flying back to London, I took the train home to Durham. My mum was waiting on the platform.

'Wow!' she said, as I walked towards her. 'I send you away blobby and you come back gorgeous!'

'Hardly.'

'You look healthy! Do you feel better?'

'In some ways. But, well, I've lots to tell you when we're home.'

As soon as I'd dumped my flight bag in the hallway, I told my mum about the reflexologist, and the wonderful hotel food, and about my digestive system and joints healing.

'Come here,' Mum said, pulling me into her arms. 'I'm thrilled you've come back so much better. You'll possibly even get back to Trinity Hall this autumn.'

I recoiled. 'Possibly? Why would you think I might not be going back to Cambridge?'

'Because you've been so ill. But I never said I didn't think you would. I said I thought you *probably* would.'

'You said possibly.'

Mum sighed. 'And there I was thinking Jon was the lawyer.' And she left me there to 'rest', this time meaning to calm down.

*

The improvements in my health on holiday quickly faded as I fell back into my old routines. The aches in my knees and elbows returned, as did my crampy bowel pains. Worse still, the glandular fever threatened a relapse.

Optimistically, I had dusted down my Cambridge files to revise the subjects I had worked on in my first year. But after reading for no more than fifteen minutes, I would 'have a thingy'. This was a phrase my mum coined for when my face swelled up until it looked like I had lost my chin – proving that her six years at med school learning medical terminology hadn't been wasted. Then, if I continued pushing myself, the colour would drain from my face and the 'blobbiness' would spread to include my eyelids.

While this was going on, my brain fog would descend and leave me feeling like I was looking through muslin. The harder I tried to fight it, the thicker the fog would become. I would also experience a strange sensation like my eyes were being pulled back into my head. When I described these symptoms to my immunologist, he would say, 'I'm sorry, I can't offer you a magic pill.' But I didn't want a magic pill, I just wanted an explanation for the weird things that were going on in my body.

I also wanted to know why my health had improved in Malta, only to deteriorate when I was back home. Was it due to my change in diet? Or the reflexology? I needed to find out. I told Mum I would like to try a full course of reflexology in Durham and to go on an elimination diet, and she said she would ask around at work for the name of a good dietician. Meanwhile, I would find a reflexologist.

It felt like we had a battle plan.

*

'Your angel is watching over you,' said Clara, the reflexologist I had tracked down through the British Association of Reflexologists. We were in my parents' living room, and as I pulled off my sock, a perfectly white feather detached itself from the material and drifted over the massage chair towards the fireplace.

'Sorry?' I asked.

'The feather. Did you not know? Often when angels visit, they leave a white feather.'

I had no idea what to say to that, but the silence was becoming awkward. 'Why?' I eventually asked.

'So you know they've been,' she said matter-of-factly, and the spiritual Lily stirred somewhere and thought, *well, maybe*.

Then the scientist Lily returned and gave the other Lily an earful for being so gullible. I climbed into the massage chair and tried my best to relax.

Just as the Maltese practitioner had done, Clara accurately diagnosed everything that was wrong with me – even obscure things like a finger I had once caught in a door, and my teeth, which had been sensitive for a couple of days. Reflexology didn't cure me though, not even after a couple of months of treatment. All the same, I decided to keep up with the sessions for many years. My oedema always improved afterwards and I'd feel temporarily less brain fogged.

As for that business with the angel, well, that was the start of a whole new story.

*

Mum found me a marvellous dietician at my local hospital,

and I was put on a strict elimination diet for two weeks. She said I might struggle eating little more than pears and rice for a whole fourteen days. I was just worried about surviving the fortnight without chocolate.

The diet proved that gluten was responsible for most of the pains in my joints and digestive system. I also suspected I had a cow's milk intolerance because small amounts made me feel nauseous and brain fogged. But these symptoms could also be caused by EBV, so I needed more evidence. I added a little more cow's milk to my diet each day to see what would happen.

One Saturday night, when Jon was visiting, I got my answer. It was suppertime, and I had just finished a bowl of rice pudding when my guts did a somersault. I had to fly to the downstairs toilet to vomit violently. And copiously. Then the diarrhoea started and… well, I will spare you the details. Fortunately, my mum was passing and heard what was going on. She pushed a bucket at me and said, 'Sit on the toilet, vomit in there.'

The smell of bleach and plastic emanating from the bucket made the nausea worse. Soon my throat was sore from retching. As if that wasn't enough, my legs suddenly became insanely itchy. When I scratched them, I felt lumps coming up through my skin. I started to feel woozy, and darkness hovered at the edges of my vision.

'Lily?' Mum called from outside. 'Are you OK?'

'I think… I'm going to faint.'

She poked her head around the door, took one look at me, then called for an emergency doctor.

I knew enough about allergic reactions to realise I was in trouble. My symptoms were escalating quickly, and it crossed my mind that the next stage could be anaphylaxis. The thought terrified me. I could hear my mum on the phone to the doctor, but what were the chances of him getting here in time?

Then as abruptly as the reaction started, it stopped. No blackout, no more vomiting, I could breathe. Relief flooded through me.

Still light-headed, I struggled to focus on Mum as she re-entered the room. She was carrying…

A *camera*? 'What are you doing?' I rasped.

'Warming up the flash.'

I almost dropped the bucket. 'Are you mad? This isn't the time to update the family album!'

'I need a few photos of those,' she said, waving a hand at the lumps on my torso and legs. 'Otherwise, how will we describe them at your next hospital appointment?'

'But I'm wearing skimpy pants!'

'I'll be showing these to your doctor, not sending them to the press.'

'Still.'

She laughed. 'You are *such* a prude!'

I waited for the rest of the speech she always rolls out at such times – where she says that medics don't see your bits like normal people do, and how after catheterising dozens of men as a junior doctor she had started to see penises like any other appendage. For once, though, she spared me the full spiel, which showed how worried she must have been.

'Where's Jon?' I asked.

'Watching the match with Dad. Don't worry, I said I'd take care of you.'

Typical. I nearly die, and the men barely take their eyes

off the game. On the other hand, perhaps this wasn't the best time for Jon to see me.

I grabbed my jeans and tried to pull them on. But I was still feeling dizzy and it proved to be a harder task than I had expected. I grasped the sink to steady myself.

'Wait!' said Mum as I had one foot halfway down a trouser leg. 'How about I get you some more respectable pants? *Then* can I take the photos?'

At my next immunology appointment, Dr Spickett and my mum pored over the photographs of my red, swollen, hive-covered body. They thought it had been a type-one allergic reaction, and to confirm it, I endured my usual bloodletting at the hands of the nurses. But the blood test came back negative, meaning I had 'merely' suffered a severe intolerance reaction. Unfortunately, it had reactivated my glandular fever. Soon I was back in bed with a fever and a moon face, and it took months of Aciclovir to make me better.

I had missed my chance to return to Cambridge. Again.

*

I was left to spend the autumn alone at home. My friends were at university, and Jon was beavering away in the City. I felt trapped. I needed to free myself from my stuffy room and reacquaint myself with the world outside. So, I would put on my big, student jumper that reminded me of cold afternoons in Cambridge labs, then set off down the drive.

At first, I set my targets low. I would challenge myself to walk the hundred or so paces to the nearest postbox just to prove that I could do it. But by the time I got there, I would be so 'out of it' that I wouldn't know if I could make it back. Then, when I did get home, I used to spread out in a star shape on the hallway carpet and stare up at the ceiling, wondering how such a short stroll could floor me like this.

Yet the next day I would go and do the same thing again.

One afternoon, I set off for my walk as usual, only to make it less than halfway to the postbox before needing to stop. I leant against a lamp post, fearing I didn't have the strength to continue. Then the strangest thing happened: I was overwhelmed by a smell of fresh flowers so strong it was like I was back in the Cambridge Botanic Garden. I looked around for the source, but there was nothing to see except passing cars and a man in an anorak smoking his life away. Certainly no florists or secret gardens nearby.

The fragrance lingered.

I watched a bus pull into its stop on the other side of the road. As it drove off again, it left a trail of diesel fumes. But nothing could mask the floral aroma.

Mystified, I gathered my strength and set off for home.

My thoughts drifted. Maybe the postbox had been a bridge too far today, but I consoled myself with the knowledge that at least I had succeeded in getting out. Ahead, a woman with two giant schnauzers emerged from the vet's surgery. As I watched the dogs drag their owner across the road, I suddenly sensed someone right behind me. After a few steps I swung around, conscious that my personal space was being invaded.

But there was no one there. Odd.

As I passed the vet's, the floral smell intensified. And whilst I could hear no footfalls, I became convinced that someone was moving up alongside me. My skin prickled. The day was still, yet I felt the air beside me… change. Glancing across, I saw nothing but empty pavement. Perhaps I should have been scared or intimidated, but instead all I felt was calm. Peaceful, even. It was as if the angel on my shoulder had stepped down for a moment.

Behind, I heard distant barks from the schnauzers. I crossed the road towards my house. Then, as I reached the drive, the smell vanished.

I opened the front door, walked into the hallway, and tried to figure out what the heck had just happened.

Chapter 8

Life continued as normal with my walks to the postbox and my visits from Jon. When Jon wasn't around, my parents kept me in good spirits. If I was having a bad day and wanted to cry on Mum's shoulder, she would calmly talk me through everything. Once, when I complained about how hard life was, she replied, 'It is absolutely *shit* at times, love. I don't know how you're coping. Let's watch *Corrie* and eat chocolate.'

You can see why she made such a good psychiatrist.

By contrast, when Dad and I noticed each other's expressions there would be no need for words. He'd be slumped in his big armchair – the one with the recliner that he never uses – and I'd go and sit on one of the arm rests, legs across him. If we did talk at all, he would sigh and say something lofty about how life sometimes throws up obstacles, but that when Plan A doesn't work out you just have to go on to Plan B, then Plan C. But you will always find happiness before you get to Plan Z. I wasn't entirely convinced.

On Saturday nights, provided I hadn't managed to persuade my parents to go out, we would settle in the lounge together and have a TV dinner – something my dad whipped up because he's a whiz in the kitchen. Mum would insist on watching *Casualty* because she's obsessed with anything medical. When she sat right back on the sofa, her slippered feet wouldn't touch the floor, and I would watch her short legs dangling over the edge.

One night, after she had spoiled the episode entirely by diagnosing everyone within the first five minutes, I said, 'You love medicine like I love science, don't you?'

'Yes!' she said, smiling.

Then not smiling. I had killed the moment completely. She looked at me with her sorrowful eyes and patted my leg. It was clear she didn't think I would make it through this illness to become the scientist trapped inside me.

I stopped watching *Casualty* soon after that. Not because of Mum, but because I spent so much time in hospitals that I couldn't face watching them on screen. In fact, I stopped watching a lot of programmes that I had once enjoyed.

'Where are you going?' my dad asked one Sunday evening as I made to leave the lounge. '*Ski Sunday* is about to start.' *Ski Sunday* was integral to my family's existence.

'I can't watch it any more, Dad. I just can't.'

I saw his look change from confusion to sadness as the realisation hit him that I would probably never ski again. Forcing a jovial tone, he said, 'Well, let's watch something else, then. We don't have to see the same thing every week, do we?'

'It's fine, Dad,' I pretended. 'I won't stop you watching skiing.' It would be like stopping Mum watching medical programmes – nothing short of cruelty. I gave him a hug and turned towards the doorway.

As I was leaving the room, Mum entered it.

'Where's she going?' she asked Dad. 'Doesn't she know *Ski Sunday* is about to start?'

*

One afternoon while I was lying in bed, Mum marched into my room and perched on the edge of my duvet. 'Seeing as you've started to embrace alternative medicine,' she said, 'have you thought about herbalism? It's using plants as medicine. There's a lady doing a talk on it at our next Rotary meeting, if you want to come.'

I pulled myself upright. 'I'd love to, if I'm well enough.'

'How well would you have to be? You just have to sit there and listen. Then we'll drive you back home.'

Comments like that used to sadden me. My parents understood my ill health better than anyone. But if they didn't realise how strenuous it was for me to get washed and dressed, then sit upright for a whole hour, what chance was there that anyone else would?

Still, a few days later I was sitting in the function room of a pub, watching a middle-aged lady wave an apple about as she boomed, 'Nature provides us with all the medicines we need!' She had a PhD in virology, so I figured she must know what she was talking about. After her speech, when I found myself sharing the hand dryer with her in the ladies', I asked her about her practice. Before my hands were fully dry I had arranged an appointment to see her.

Yet, the following Saturday afternoon, as I walked down the quaint stone path to her house, I felt uneasy. I disliked the insular approach of many mainstream doctors, but a lot of alternative medicine seemed like witchcraft to me. So, when I entered her house and saw a black cat walking along the back of her sofa, I half looked for the broomstick to go with it.

The herbalist led me through to her conservatory. It reminded me of the botany laboratories at Cambridge with its potted plants, stacks of books, pipettes and glass bottles. I fidgeted in my chair as I relayed my symptoms, then poked out my tongue when instructed. Half an hour later, I left her house with a brown bottle filled with a viscous liquid that smelt like something you would spit out at the dentist's.

I took the medicine twice daily, along with the molasses she prescribed for my 'anaemia'. (I never was anaemic, but I can understand why the herbalist thought I was because my post-viral pallor is quite striking.) My health began to improve: my oedema drained, my glands got smaller, and my head felt clearer. I had evidently underestimated the power of plants. The scientist in me got excited and wanted to know more. I asked the herbalist to send me a list of the herbs I was taking so I could find out about their properties.

But when I received that list and started researching the herbs on it, I was dismayed to discover that some of them were known to worsen, or even cause, auto-immune diseases. I already had hypothyroidism, arthritis, and possibly coeliac disease, and the last thing I wanted was to add another illness to my list. So, I stopped swallowing the sticky brown liquor, and the glandular fever symptoms worsened again.

I couldn't win.

*

The start of the next academic year was fast approaching. By August it was obvious I would be too ill to return to Cambridge that autumn. I asked college for another year out, and they agreed. In Durham, people told me I needed to start mixing with other people and to spend more time studying so I was 'ready' for university the following year. I signed up at my local college for once-a-week classes in English Literature. Surely my health could manage *that*.

Apparently not. In my first term, I attended barely half the classes. And whilst I enjoyed the writing, I wasn't so keen on sharing a classroom with the other students' germs. My battle against glandular fever had left me particularly vulnerable to catching other infections. So, as sure as dessert follows main course, whenever I went to college I would come down with a bug and be forced to miss the following lesson, if not the one after that too. And even when I succeeded in dodging the bugs, I'd still end up having to spend the next six days in bed recovering from the class.

Jon had finished his traineeship at his law firm and had always intended to travel before starting life as a qualified solicitor. He wanted to go on safari to Kenya, then visit Egypt and dive in the Red Sea – plans he had made with a friend of his a few years before. But when the time came to pay for the tickets, his friend pulled out, and suddenly Jon wasn't sure if he should go.

'I don't think I want to go anyway,' he said on the phone to me one evening.

'Why? You've been planning this for *years*.'

'But then I met someone as… special as you,' he said, in a rare declaration of his feelings.

I told him in my usual overzealous fashion that this was

his dream, and that neither a fickle friend nor a burst of sentimentality should take that away from him.

Afterwards, people told me I was mad to let my boyfriend travel alone for a month. But what made me determined he should go (apart from my previously expressed belief that you have to live your life while you still have the health) was that I knew deep down I would never be able to do those things with him. I wanted him to try them now and come back choosing the settled life with the invalid, rather than not do them, and perhaps one day resent me for it.

Shortly after he left, I answered the phone to a soft male voice barely audible over the crackle of interference. It was Jon calling from a hut in Kenya.

'I have to be quick,' he said. 'I had to bribe a local to use his phone, and his expression tells me he wants it back. I just wanted to say thank you for making me come here. I love you.'

And then it cut off.

I floated through that EBV relapse on a cloud of happiness.

*

While Jon was on his travels, I had extra time alone to think. I realised my illness was making me look at the world in a different light. At one extreme, I watched the stressed-out businesspeople on the trains to London, banging on their laptops and talking curtly on their phones. Cardiac arrests waiting to happen, most of them. I hoped they had someone at home who made them realise what was important.

At the other extreme were the Kosovan refugees I saw on TV. At this time, the war in the Balkans was going on, and every night there were images of thousands of stranded people living in tents. Children wandered around crying, looking for parents who were possibly lost, probably killed. I tried to extrapolate from my own ordeal and imagine how these people must be feeling. But their suffering was worlds apart from mine. I decided I had to do something for them.

The next day I contacted my church. On behalf of Samaritan's Purse, the priest was collecting shoeboxes filled with toys and essentials. Determined to play my part, I raided our wardrobes for shoeboxes, then went to the local shops for supplies. People heard what I was doing and began dropping off donated goods in carrier bags. It was too much for me physically, yet it helped me on an emotional level. No one could alleviate my situation, but I could help to make things better for others.

One hundred and eight. That's how many shoeboxes I managed to put together thanks to people's generosity. As I slid into my next relapse, I thought at least this one had been worth it. But four months later, with the virus still rampant, I wasn't so convinced. Mum banned me from doing more than a dozen boxes the following year. I took twelve to be her opening bid and got her up to thirty.

In the midst of my shoebox endeavours, Jon was due back from his trip. He called me from Egypt to enthuse about his scuba diving and to check I would be in London to meet him when he returned. I mopped my brow and assured him I would be there. Mum said I was crazy even to consider going, but a week later I was on the train with a nearly normal temperature.

As I was boiling the kettle in his apartment, I saw Jon's sunburnt face and floppy bleached fringe at the kitchen window. I still remember the elation in his expression when he clocked my face. He rushed inside, then dropped his oversized backpack and swung me round.

Sometimes I feel so lucky with my loved ones, I think I'm greedy for wanting better health from life too.

*

Let me get one thing straight: I was gaining some perspective, along with some much-needed compassion and understanding. But don't think for one minute that I had dropped the Cambridge dream. Ultimately, I was going to be a brilliant academic.

I still had a way to go on the humility front.

But the shoebox relapse had set me back a long way. The months ticked by, yet my wretched virus was going nowhere. I turned twenty-two, and it was depressing to think I had now been ill for almost five years. I was clearly too unwell to return to Cambridge in October, so I asked my college for another year out and they agreed.

However, that December my tutor phoned me and asked how likely I thought it was that I would recover enough to start the following year. He said that as I had been so long out of college now, it might be an idea to repeat the first year to refresh my knowledge. And as they had a glut of applications that year, they needed to know if they should save a place for me or allow someone else to have it.

I remember that call as if it were yesterday, standing in the cold hallway while my mum passed back and forth across the landing, gathering her belongings for the gym. It's strange how our hearts speak the truth when we're put on the spot and our heads don't have time to interfere. Up to then, my brain hadn't entertained the idea of never being well enough to return. But as I stood there, I thought of all the sixth formers who had painstakingly filled in their Cambridge application forms. They would be waiting at home right now, hoping for a yes just as I had five years ago. And whilst *my* odds of recovery might be slim, they still had the chance to become the scientist I wanted to be.

'I think I should officially leave and let someone else take my place,' I made myself say. Although the words crushed me.

There was silence for a moment, then my tutor asked quietly, 'What will you do?'

'Get better,' I said. 'Then one day I might write a book.'

That was the first I knew about that too. Like I say, sometimes our hearts have the answers.

*

I was in freefall. All those years of striving towards the big career had come to a dead end. For most of my life I had thought of myself as a scientific researcher in the making. Now I didn't know what I was or where I was going. I felt like a compass with a permanently spinning needle. I needed it to stop turning and point where I should go. I spent days trying to make sense of what had happened – days fighting through a feverish brain fog, searching for the way forward. The book idea was pushed into a corner of my mind because I refused to give up on being a scientist just yet.

Then one day my fever abated, and I sat bolt upright in bed. *Right, that's it*, I thought.

It was time for Plan B.

Chapter 9

So, I wasn't going to graduate from Cambridge, but that didn't mean I couldn't still have a career. Cambridge life had been a dawn-to-dusk frenzy of lectures, practicals and tutorials, with more lectures at weekends. But what if I applied to another university that offered a better work-rest balance? Then I wouldn't have to recover completely, just partly. Partly was far more achievable.

I focused on the University of York, not only because it had a great reputation, but also because it was close to home in case something went wrong. I went to one of its open days and liked everything about the place: the campus, the course content, the lecturers I spoke to. And as quickly as that, my mind was made up. I couldn't wait to start.

Obviously, my health would need to improve first. My mum, having already found me the best immunologist in the North of England, wondered if there was anyone who could give a second opinion on how to make me better. Dr Spickett recommended an immunologist in London.

So, the following month I found myself sitting in the waiting room of the immunology department of a London hospital. It was such a different place from the hospital I was used to back home. In the waiting room at Newcastle, there was a buzz as the friendly nurses shuttled patients back and forth for their weigh-ins and blood tests. And the patients looked *healthy*. They hid their immune disorders so well it made me wonder if I'd taken a wrong turn on the way to the department.

But in that huge, bleak waiting room in London, everyone looked at death's door. The surly receptionist slapped a clipboard on the counter and demanded I fill in the questionnaire, then sighed when I said I didn't have a pen on me. My dad hastily got his own out before she collapsed under the weight of her world-weariness.

The chairs were arranged in a large square around a table. Pale, skinny people were scattered here and there: a girl about my age, asleep in a wheelchair; two men holding hands staring worriedly at the floor; and finally two women in their seventies – one looking morose, the other nattering about the granary loaf she'd bought earlier at the supermarket. Hers was the only voice in this desolate room.

Obviously, it was just a matter of time before my dad added his voice to hers; any sense of gloom and he was always quick to dispel it with his chit-chat. I remember one occasion when we were in an Indian restaurant, waiting for our takeaway biryani to arrive, and he started singing along to 'The Lady in Red' on the radio. He was even clicking his fingers. No way was I risking a repeat of that here. I turned to him and warned him that I was already feeling stressed, so a moment like that now might tip me over the edge. Then I relaxed, confident I had poured water on the kindling before any sparks could land.

Alas, it wasn't to be.

The appointments were running late. I hadn't eaten for several hours, and my low blood sugar had put a tremor in my hands. Dad started slapping his pockets in a hunt for snacks. Finding them empty, he scanned the waiting room for something consumable. And then… *noooooooo*.

I could see what was about to happen, but there was nothing I could do to stop it. On the table with the magazines was a basket of… coloured packets. Dad reached for the basket and placed it on his lap.

'What are these?' he asked.

I grabbed at his elbow to make him stop, but he ignored me.

'I need my glasses,' he said, 'but I left them in the car.' So, he picked up a red packet, squinted, then read aloud: 'Strawberry flavoured? Oh. Ha! Ha ha!'

He didn't actually *say* the word 'condom'. He didn't need to. The entire waiting room watched me as I squirmed. The two guys sat transfixed; the talkative old lady sniggered, probably delighted she now had a better story to tell her friends than the one about granary bread. Only two people remained oblivious to what was going on: the girl asleep in the wheelchair, and my mum, engrossed in a medical magazine. But as Dad struggled to suppress his laughter, Mum lifted her nose out of the BMJ and asked, 'What have I missed?'

'I'll tell you later,' I whispered.

'Tell me now.'

'No! Later.'

'Lily, I've obviously missed something important.' All eyes in the room were on us, and Dad's laughter was threatening to bubble over. 'What just happened?'

So, my dad re-enacted the whole episode and I was forced

to endure the ordeal again. By the time I was called into my appointment, I was so flushed I nearly looked healthy.

In terms of the EBV relapses, there was nothing new the immunologist could test for or suggest. But he wondered if some of my facial swelling could be due to allergy.[2] He suggested I try a course of antihistamine tablets to see if they helped.

Mum was worried I would refuse to take them. I had already said no to various medicines over the years – things that were said to boost the 'energy' of people with ME/CFS. But I had only turned down these drugs previously because I didn't feel tired, and I wasn't prepared to take medication to alleviate a symptom I didn't have. The immunologist told me to think of the antihistamines as an experiment; if they helped, then allergy was a factor in my illness. If they didn't, then I could come off them.

So, I started taking the pills, and after a few days I improved, especially in terms of my brain fog. Antihistamines weren't going to produce the big recovery I was hoping for, but at least they gave me the headspace to think once more.

*

Around this time, I started to become really interested in the health effects of foods. On a good day, I would drive

---

2 One of the theories surrounding ME/CFS that has been triggered by glandular fever is that the immune system doesn't 'reset' itself properly after tackling the EBV. The result is that the patient is left susceptible to things the immune system would normally fight (bugs), and overreacting to things it shouldn't be attacking (allergens). It was, therefore, possible that my continued facial swelling was due to an allergic response rather than the EBV itself, which is why the tablets were worth a try. The immunologist had already successfully treated two ME/CFS patients this way.

into town and wander up Saddler Street to Waterstones so I could browse its nutrition section. The first book I bought from that store was a guide called *Foods That Harm, Foods That Heal*. Dozens more books were to follow. Some had a medical or a biological slant; others took a holistic approach.

I have loved food since I was a six-year-old with ribbons in my hair, sitting on the kitchen worktop beating eggs for a chocolate cake. Nowadays, I am more interested in the idea that you can alter the chemical reactions inside you with the molecules you swallow. Sometimes I would ask my mum to track down a medical paper that was referred to in my books, about things like the effects of zinc on the body or the role of essential fatty acids in health. If the London immunologist had been right when he suggested my immune system hadn't 'reset' properly (and that certainly would explain why I caught every bug going, as well as why I felt better on antihistamines), then I would just have to change my diet and supplement regime to try to shift it back towards normal.

I made simple changes at first: increasing the quantity of foods and drinks that have antiviral properties (like cruciferous vegetables, garlic and green tea) and consuming fewer foods that suppress the immune system (like sugar). In fact, it was doubly important for me to cut down on sugar because whenever I ate a lot of it, my body became incredibly sore to the touch. No doctor could tell me why. I later found out that EBV can alter your glucose metabolism, which may hold the key to an explanation.

The dietary changes kick-started my recovery, and I woke one day to find I had a normal temperature and visible cheekbones. My next blood test showed that my IgM antibodies were temporarily undetectable. It felt like I had won the battle… for now.

Having been bed bound for the best part of six years, I decided it was time to start building up my muscles again. When I was well enough, I used to go with Mum to the beauty salon up the road. After collapsing onto one of their toning tables (they're like exercise machines for people who don't want to do any, you know, exercise), I would be shunted along the row until I came out the other end strong and trim. (I wish!)

Unfortunately, the experience did me as much harm as good. Maybe the tables helped me rebuild some muscle mass, but the effort of regularly pulling on my gym gear and dragging myself to the salon was more than my health could handle.

No doubt the physical effect they had on me – turning me paler and blobby again – wasn't quite what Mum had been hoping for. Still, I hadn't realised how much she was struggling with the slowness of my recovery until she came into my bedroom one wintry afternoon to find me huddled under my duvet. She folded down the top of the quilt so she could see my face.

'Lily,' she said, 'I haven't been entirely honest with you these last few months. You know when I go to the gym?'

'Yes?'

'Well. The thing is… I don't always go to the gym.'

I gasped. 'Are you seeing another man?'

'Don't be ridiculous!'

'Then where have you been going?'

'You know the Coal Hole pub?'

'Yes.'

'I go there.'

''To drink?'

'Ha! No. To cry.' She looked out of the window. Sleet was catching on the glass and sliding down to the sill. 'I don't actually go into the pub. I just park in the lay-by outside. Do you know where I mean?'

I nodded, not taking my eyes off her. So that had been her mode of release – her way of coping with my illness. I felt sick with guilt.

'I didn't want you to know,' she continued. 'But I had to tell you now because it explains the next bit.'

My heart was hammering. What on earth could be coming next? What was worse than my mother weeping in lay-bys?

She looked back at me. 'I've been wondering how I can get out of this hole. I think part of the problem is that I'm struggling to be your mum, your doctor and your... counsellor.'

I saw now where this was going. 'I don't need a counsellor.'

'I just thought, if you had someone else to talk to other than me, I'd be better able to do the mothering bit.'

'I've got lots of friends to talk to.'

'Who don't understand what you're going through.'

'And I've got Jon.'

'Who is your normality – whom you want to share the good times with. I'm thinking of someone who could take over some of my role.'

I eyed her suspiciously. 'Like who?'

'Well, I've been putting the feelers out—'

'Of course you have.'

'And I've found a really good... well, she's a psychologist

by profession. But before you jump down my throat, let me say that she's bright and friendly, and that she's used to working with young women. What do you think? Would you see her? For me?'

She looked desperate, yet she must have known I would agree. I would walk across broken glass for her, and, quite frankly, this would hurt a lot less. 'Of course I'll see her,' I said, despite feeling this would just be another way of wasting my health.

Her smile extinguished my reservations.

*

I was never sure whether Mum genuinely needed me to talk to someone for her sake, or whether it was a ploy to make me agree to counselling. Whatever the case, the sessions turned out to be fun. Anna, the psychologist, was the sort of person I'd have had as a friend in a different life, so it was easy opening up to her.

I asked her if she could do cognitive behavioural therapy (CBT) with me because I had read it was effective for people with ME/CFS. But she said I didn't need it. She said I could *be* a CBT therapist because I had such a positive outlook on my condition.

There were other things I brought up with Anna. For example, since leaving Cambridge I had had nightmares every night. During the day I knew I still had everything to live for, starting with the University of York in a matter of months. Yet, once I fell asleep, dreadful things used to happen. In the 'milder' nightmares, I would be on a long journey, and my car would break down or my train would derail – clear representations of how I saw my life. But in the worst ones, I would be physically attacked: shot, knifed, or raped. Sometimes, after I woke up, I would run to turn on the light and stand there in the glare, panting.

Then I'd tell myself to get a grip and go back to bed.

Only to fall into another nightmare.

Anna told me to keep a dream diary, and to make a note of my physical state each day, especially my temperature. We found that the worst nightmares coincided with when I had a fever. My body was under attack, so my sleeping mind portrayed me under attack too.

'So, I'm not as screwed up as I feared,' I said.

'You're not screwed up at all,' replied Anna. 'Your brain is just trying to make sense of what you are going through.'

I gained a lot from those sessions. Anna gave me logical explanations for things I had previously considered to be irrational – not just the nightmares, but also the feelings of insecurity. For instance, around this time my parents drove me to Newcastle to do some Christmas shopping. It was a while since I had been able to get out of the house, and as I walked through Eldon Garden Shopping Centre, I started to feel anxious. People rushed by, knocking me with their bags. Plus, the noise, the chatter, the blaring Christmas music – it was too much for someone who was used to the silence of her sick house. I began to panic.

My mum, unaware of my feelings, said, 'Do you want to go around with us, or would you rather shop alone?'

The thought of being by myself scared me so much there was only one thing I could do.

'I think I should shop alone,' I said. Because I knew I had to face this head-on.

So, we parted, and I walked into John Lewis. As I headed past the cosmetics counters and towards the escalator, I kept telling myself to calm down, and by the time I was on the second floor I had dispelled my demons. But I'm glad that experience happened. I'm glad I had a taste of what my illness could have done to me if I hadn't made every effort to get out when I could.

I told Anna about the episode, and she drew a graph for me showing how events in my life would have caused anxiety, and how that anxiety builds up. Sometimes it peaks when you least expect it. That really helped me, because when I feel anxious now, I picture that graph and make myself relax. It keeps me grounded in an otherwise bizarre existence.

*

My counselling course finished just before the new millennium. Jon came to stay for New Year's Eve, along with my brother and his partner. Mum bought us tickets for her gym's party. There was no way I would be healthy enough to stay the whole time, so instead Jon and I arranged to come later.

In those days I had to cut corners whenever I went out, so the getting-ready bit didn't end up being all I was able to do. I no longer bothered with hair conditioner because I needed a long lie-down just to recover from rinsing out the shampoo. Eyeshadow and lipstick went the same way; I embraced the 'natural' look. But that night, I wore a sparkly dress and even put on some make-up, despite the fact that no amount of foundation could hide my pallor.

I managed one dance and spent the rest of the night recovering from it while the drunken hordes giggled and sashayed into tables. Then just before midnight, everyone moved outside for the fireworks.

As the clock struck twelve, I was overwhelmed with sadness. Jon hugged me, his chin resting on my head. I felt loved and protected, but I also felt lost, because I had contracted glandular fever in 1994 and here I was – six years later – still ill and back on the Aciclovir. I started to cry.

'I hope those are happy tears,' Jon whispered.

I had to be honest with him. Over the boom and crash of fireworks, I told him how miserable I was that my life was amounting to nothing.

He looked stunned. Then he stared into my eyes and said calmly, 'Lily, one day you will set the world alight.'

His words moved me. Not because they were true (though I was willing to give it my best shot, dammit), but because it struck me that he was the only person who always had faith in me – who saw me as me, not as the illness.

So as my tears turned into genuinely happy ones, I discovered a new resolve.

New millennium. It was time to get my life back on track.

*

'We need another holiday,' said Jon a few weeks later. 'Shall we book one for the spring?'

Spring seemed like a good idea because it was months away; there was plenty of time to get better. I was going to need that time too, since I had started the millennium as I'd finished the last one: stuck in an immunological rut. We booked flights to Barcelona along with a stay in an apartment in the hills.

By the time spring came, I was off the Aciclovir. But as I boarded the plane to Spain, my deathly white face was still enough to put the frighteners on the cabin crew – so much so that a flight attendant asked me if I had a medical certificate proving I was well enough to fly!

It's strange thinking back to my early holidays with Jon. He remembers watching sunsets together and setting off in hire cars to explore ancient ruins, whereas I remember looking for places to sit down. I exaggerate slightly. Those trips helped keep me sane, and I was relieved for the chance to escape from home. But when you are as ill as I was, a holiday can amount to little more than a new bed to lie down in. And on the times you are able to go sightseeing, you use up so much health travelling that you can't appreciate whatever it is you've gone to visit.

In Barcelona that time, I hauled myself around some Roman remains before dragging myself to Las Ramblas, where I got upset about some emaciated guinea pigs that were for sale. But then I had to head back while I still had the strength to stand. To this day, people say to me, 'You went to Barcelona and you didn't see the Sagrada Familia? Or the Olympic Village? Why not?' And I don't even try to explain that my life with Jon is full of these compromises – that I am just grateful to get away at all.

Back in our apartment, I sent Jon off to the golf course while I arranged a reflexology session in the health centre downstairs. In Malta, my treatment at the hands of the all-diagnosing therapist had proved hugely beneficial, if a bit surreal, and I was hoping for more of the same on this holiday. Little was I to know that the strangeness was about to get dialled up to a whole new level.

The session started off well. The petite, curly haired reflexologist lit fragranced candles around the therapy room while I lay listening to the otherworldly music floating from her cassette player. I closed my eyes and began to relax.

Abruptly, the reflexologist stopped the Gregorian chanting and put on some opera music. And not the relaxing sort either, if there is such a thing. Instead, I was treated to the sound of a woman seemingly singing her way through her own murder. Next, the reflexologist whipped off my socks and pulled each of my toes so firmly, they cracked. Then she started massaging my feet. Except this wasn't like any other massage I had experienced. It felt more like she was trying to push her thumbs through my soles. I gritted my teeth and considered asking her to reduce the pressure, but before I could do so, she broke into song.

Startled, I opened my eyes and looked at her. Her eyes were focused on mine, her voice filled with emotion as she sang along to the opera music. Sang very well, actually, but still.

I gave her a hesitant smile.

Her expression didn't change.

I tried a cough to check she hadn't fallen into some sort of trance, but perhaps she had done just that, because she didn't acknowledge me at all. I realised she was not so much looking *at* me as *through* me.

I shut my eyes so I couldn't see her.

Eventually the session ended, and I was relieved to find myself still alive. The reflexologist turned off the opera tape and transformed back into a normal forty-something-year-old as if the oddball stuff hadn't even happened. I hurriedly put on my socks and trainers and made to leave. But as I passed the reflexologist, she caught my arm. Her look held so much warmth and compassion, I thought she was going to cry.

'I not often treat someone like you,' she said. 'You are very… special. I not know the English. How you say? Sensitive? Intuit…?'

'Intuitive?'

'Yes. But more than that. Si… Sike…'

'Psychic?'

'Yes!' she said again, pleased that I understood.

'No,' I said, looking frantically for the exit. 'I'm really not.'

'Yes, you are. But you think too much.' She tapped her head. 'You stop all that thinking, then you see spirits.'

I resolved to continue 'thinking too much'.

The reflexologist clutched my hand in both of hers. 'I feel blessed I met you. I wish you luck with… everything.'

Smiling awkwardly, I retrieved my hand and fled.

Back in England, I told my mum and she appeared interested.

'Do you believe all this psychic lark?' I asked her.

Mum's expression gave nothing away. 'What do you believe?'

*

Weeks later, I was lying in bed, recovering from the holiday and unable to sleep, when what I can only describe as a column of bright light appeared at my bedside. I shut my eyes. This was either hypnagogia (the state between wake and sleep when the mind can do strange things) or it was something from on high. Either way, I wanted it to go away fast, so I asked it politely to leave. Then I reopened my eyes.

The shaft of light remained.

'And just for the record, I am *not* psychic,' I muttered.

Still there.

I closed my eyes again and turned over in bed so that I faced the other way. My anxiety levels were rising, so I pictured my psychologist's graph and forced myself to think of relaxing times – like sharing the sunlounger with Jon on our balcony in Spain and laughing at his cringey jokes. It must have worked because the next thing I knew, it was morning.

After persuading myself that the light had been a trick of the mind, I went downstairs and told my mum about it. I thought she would be amazed, or intrigued, or offer some convoluted psychiatric explanation. Instead, she simply nodded as if I'd told her I was having cornflakes for breakfast.

Then she asked, 'How did it make you feel?'

'Freaked out!'

But it was odd how easily she had accepted it. Had she witnessed things like this herself? It felt like I was learning something new about my mother every day.

Chapter 10

It was August, and I was nowhere near healthy enough to start my degree at York the following month. I was barely managing to attend a third of my English night classes, and they were only once a week. At York I would be expected to be at lectures every weekday.

It was so demoralising. It wasn't just York or being ill for six years. It was the fact that I didn't have the health to support myself. Being ill was proving to be surprisingly expensive with all the costly dietary supplements and alternative therapy sessions. Maybe if I got some financial independence, the rest would follow?

So, I decided to apply for disability benefit. I wasn't sure where to start. I contacted the Job Centre, but instead of helping, they gave me forms for the wrong benefit. Unaware of this, I wasted all my good days filling them in.

Then I relapsed from all the writing.

Months later, when my health finally picked up, I tried again. I contacted the Department of Social Security (DSS, as it then was) to ask what benefit I should be receiving. They told me it was called Severe Disablement Allowance and sent me a form that posed questions like whether I could feed myself with a fork and go to the toilet unaided. This 'one size fits all' form was for people with all kinds of disabilities, but there was no place for me to convey my particular problems. So, when I was called for a medical at an assessment centre in town a few weeks later, I was pleased because I thought it would give me a chance to explain my case.

The guy doing the assessment was a decrepit, retired GP who kept stroking his long grey beard as he asked me questions about Cambridge. I had brought in a letter from my immunologist explaining the seriousness of my illness. But the assessor refused to even look at it. Apparently, he knew my condition better than the foremost expert on immune disorders in the Northeast. He asked me questions such as, 'Can you stretch your arms in the air?' and 'Are you able to touch your toes?' He also told me to strip down to my underwear so he could measure my thighs.

I left feeling very misunderstood. At that time, people with ME/CFS were largely considered malingerers. And let's face it, my thigh measurements weren't going to prove otherwise.

A couple of weeks later I received a letter from the DSS saying the doctor considered me well enough to work because I was 'alert, coherent… talking freely with good eye contact and appearing cheerful'. In a different setting, these comments would be nice to hear, but this was a medical report. It felt like my efforts to explain my illness had been dismissed or even used against me.

They weren't going to get rid of me that easily. This was war.

The letter stated I could appeal the decision if I filled in yet another form. I sent it off, but I never got an appeal date despite constantly chasing it up. I went to the Citizens Advice Bureau for help, but there was nothing they could do. The volunteer, a kind man in his seventies, had limited knowledge of the appeals process and absolutely no understanding of my illness. I decided to up the stakes, so I tracked down my local MP. He was doing an open surgery in a local pit village, and I soon found myself explaining to him how disgracefully sufferers of my illness were treated.

Within a few days, I was given a date for a tribunal hearing. Imagine that.

I planned to go to the tribunal alone since both my parents had work commitments on the morning in question. That didn't bother me, though, because whilst my body may have been a wreck, my feisty streak was doing just fine. I researched online the criteria for the benefit I'd been refused, and as far as I was concerned I satisfied every one of them. The DSS didn't have a leg to stand on.

My parents weren't quite so confident. They had asked around about appeal tribunals and had been told I would be cut into strips if I went in without representation. So, my mum arranged for me to speak to a man called Ken who was a shining light at Durham council's welfare rights department.

The evening before the tribunal, the phone rang. It was Ken.

'Just to let you know, things probably won't go our way tomorrow,' he said.

I was floored. 'Why?'

'Because the doctor assessed you as being thirty per cent disabled, and you have to be at least eighty per cent to receive the benefit. At tribunals, they might make up a deficit of ten or twenty per cent. But not fifty.'

So, a doddering ex-GP takes my pulse, measures my

thighs, and picks a number out of thin air that governs the entire validity of my claim? Where was the logic in that?

When I put this to Ken, he sighed. 'I know,' he said. 'But that's just how it is.' He asked me to come along half an hour before the appeal started so we could go over my case. Then he ended the conversation with, 'Anyway, just be prepared to lose.'

Well, I intended to win.

*

My dad managed to reorganise his diary so he could come to my tribunal after all. Sitting in the waiting area that morning, I felt ready to set the world to rights. My dad told me not to look too animated.

'Ill people can still look animated,' I protested.

'Yes, but they don't look as ill as people who don't.'

So, I practised looking lacklustre while we waited for Ken to turn up.

When he arrived five minutes later, I was surprised to find he was enthusiastic, efficient and eager for the fight. I think I was a surprise to him too. He had seen my medical history and immunologist's report, but he hadn't appreciated how ill I was. As I chatted to him about my daily routine and the months spent in bed with EBV, he seemed genuinely moved. I could tell he was on my side. The question was whether I could get the panel to understand too.

Finally, we were called into a large, cold room that smelt of furniture polish. A lawyer, a doctor and a clerk sat across a long table from me, my dad and Ken. By this time, my health was deteriorating rapidly, but I hoped the panellists would see this, and that it would strengthen my case. They asked me in-depth questions about my life and the things that made me better or worse, about if and how I tested my limits, and about whether I thought my condition was improving. Then the doctor examined me and said my glands were enormous. I said if he thought they were big now, he should try feeling them on a bad day.

At the end, Ken stood up and did such a stirring summary of my case it could have been lifted straight from *L.A. Law*. 'This is a very ill young woman,' he concluded, 'who was a happy, healthy student with an excellent career ahead of her. A woman who has been hit by an illness that leaves her disabled over ninety per cent of the time. Lily, would you like to summarise your life before the illness? How does it compare with your life now?'

That threw me momentarily. I hadn't expected to have to contribute again, and it felt like my next words could make or break the case. I hesitated, trying to think of how best to answer, and conscious that all eyes were on me. I cleared my throat and said, 'Before my illness, I was set to be a research scientist. I was on five different sports teams, played the viola, had a big network of friends. Now, I just… breathe.'

There was silence in the room. The panellists stared at me. Had I overplayed my hand? I had said only how things were, but did they believe me? I scanned their faces for clues, yet they might have been poker players for how little their expressions revealed. My dad stared meaningfully at them across the table, then noticed I was looking at him and tried to turn away so I wouldn't see the tears in his eyes.

Too late.

We were asked to leave the room while the panel

discussed my case. Standing in the lobby, Ken, Dad and I had a stilted conversation in which we pretended to be happy to leave the decision to fate now. When we were finally called back in, I thought I detected a hint of a smile on the doctor's face. Certainly, I was being viewed with kindness. But did this mean I had won, or was he merely preparing me for bad news? My eyes scanned the papers on the desk in front of them and then I spotted something unmistakable: a great big eighty per cent handwritten in Biro. If they had agreed I was eighty per cent disabled that would mean I was entitled to the benefit. The lawyer saw I had clocked their sheet and confirmed that was indeed their decision.

For all that I was feeling dreadful, I had a skip in my step as I left the building. I had made each of the panellists understand ME/CFS! Maybe somewhere down the line that would benefit another sufferer. Seeing my illness recognised as a disability also made me feel that there was justice in the world after all. My principal conviction in life – that if you are honest and strong and fight for what you believe in, you will get there in the end – still held true. That was important to me in an existence where most of my other beliefs had been shattered.

My entitlement to disability benefit was regularly reassessed, and in the following years I had to go to several medicals and one more tribunal. But the assessments became more geared to all aspects of disability, and I found it easier to explain my illness to subsequent, more sympathetic health professionals.

I never had my thighs measured again.

*

I had a small income. Now I had to rebuild my life. Jon was determined to find places that would keep alive the scientist in me.

'I've thought of somewhere I can take you tomorrow,' he said when I was next in London.

I prayed that it didn't require much walking.

The next morning, we drove into the Kent countryside with the sun shining and the latest R.E.M. album booming out of his car's speakers. I looked across at Jon and he flashed a smile back.

'We're here,' he said as we approached a village.

I strained to read a road sign in the distance. 'No way!' I shrieked. 'Downe! We're going to Down House, aren't we?'

'Well done, Sherlock,' said Jon, evidently pleased at my reaction.

Down House is a Grade One listed building where Charles Darwin lived when he wrote *On the Origin of Species*. Its squeaky floorboards and musty air were reminiscent of many English Heritage properties, but its rooms provoked feelings that caught me unaware. Darwin had a chronic illness that went undiagnosed his entire life. In the study where he worked, there was a chamber pot behind a folding screen where he would rush to vomit when his condition overcame him. But he never let his fatigue or his digestive problems stop him from researching and writing. He dealt with his symptoms and carried on. It was all so heroic, yet so tragic.

I get annoyed at suggestions that his symptoms were those of a hypochondriac. Long after his death, people would say that he couldn't have been truly sick because he was animated and excitable. It reminded me of my dad telling me not to look animated at my tribunal – as if ill people aren't allowed to stay positive. In 2014, a Channel Four documentary tested Darwin's DNA and found genes for Crohn's disease, an illness which would explain all his symptoms. But was it fair to brand him a hypochondriac before that, just because no one could come up with a diagnosis?

Jon squeezed my hand in an attempt to rouse me from my reverie. 'Come out and do the Sandwalk with me.'

The Sandwalk was the path around the house where Darwin took his daily stroll. So, we left behind the families with their hyperactive children doing interactive displays and headed outside. As the wind rustled the trees, I was awash with emotions. I needed answers about my own illness, and I needed them *now*, not after my death like poor Darwin. Plus, I still wanted to be a scientist despite my illness. If Darwin could manage to juggle his work with his illness, why couldn't I?

*

Back in Durham, I decided to give my science career one last chance. Soon, I was convalescing in bed with a pile of shiny university brochures. Experience had shown me that I wasn't up to a full-time degree. Fine. Where could I study part-time? I discovered that the University of Leeds offered part-time degrees spread over six years rather than three. So I filled in an application form and applied to attend the university's open day.

That open day was probably the first time I felt old. I was a whole twenty-three years of age, while the majority of the people around me were seventeen. I went to talks on biology, chemistry and part-time studying. But I also wanted to attend the talk for students with disabilities, so I consulted my crumpled campus map and set off towards the venue. I was about to enter the building when the attendant, an overenthusiastic graduate in jeans and a blazer, gave a little cough and said, 'Sociology is next door.'

I was confused. 'But I want to go to disability rights,' I said. 'Is that not here?'

'Oh, sorry,' he said, his voice losing all authority. 'It's just you look...'

Well, I was all ears. I looked *what*?

'You don't look... I mean you look so...'

There was an awkward moment while my curiosity to find out how I appeared to a stranger battled with my wish to put him out of his misery. Soon he was beetroot, and I couldn't let it go on any longer, so I said, 'I don't look disabled, no.'

And I gave him a reassuring smile before moving on.

The University of Leeds was a great place for people with disabilities. Provided I was well enough to attend most of my lectures, the staff said they would tape-record the ones I missed. They would also give me a Dictaphone so I could record any lectures if I wasn't well enough to write notes. They really seemed to understand ME/CFS.

Afterwards, as Jon and I walked hand in hand back to his car, I couldn't stop chattering about all I had found out.

I could do this.

*

But that visit triggered a reactivation of my EBV. Several weeks later, back on high-dose Aciclovir, I was lying in bed when my mum suddenly called out, 'Who's up for a trip to Ireland?'

She had just got off the phone to one of her many brothers. Mum was born and raised in Ireland, and her family was planning to descend on Kilkenny for a big reunion. My first reaction was that I was too ill to travel. But everyone else was going – my brother and his partner, my grandma from Dublin, various uncles and cousins from all over Ireland. Plus, I had hardly seen these people since I fell ill. What if I *never* recovered enough to travel?

'I'll come,' I said.

Mum nearly passed out with pleasure.

On the ferry to Dublin, it was all I could do to stay upright. To make matters worse, a guy doing magic tricks in the passenger lounge kept descending on me, making it impossible for me to rest. I didn't mean to shoot him a death stare – it just popped out. But when my mum saw it, she told me to be pleasant when he next came over. That was all the encouragement he needed, and he chose me as his assistant for the card tricks. We hadn't even reached the Emerald Isle, and I was already suffering.

In Kilkenny, my mum's family seemed to have booked half the hotel we were staying at. I hadn't seen some of them for years, so I couldn't wait to catch up on their news. But with my aching body and fogged-out head, I struggled to chat. That evening, when we gathered in the bar for a meal, I found myself wedged between two oldies, picking at a salmon salad. I desperately wanted to burrow myself away in an eiderdown quilt, but I think eyebrows would have been raised if I'd dragged one down to the bar.

Everyone was nattering and laughing, and I did enough

of that too so as not to stand out. But physically, I was sinking. My throat was so sore, it hurt to talk. As I dissolved my Aciclovir in my glass of mineral water, I thought about how great it would be to attend social occasions with the health to actually enjoy them.

After the meal, I continued mingling for as long as I could. Everyone was so sweet, but at half past nine I slipped away to my lovely bed so I could lie down and wait for my aches to dissipate. That's right, five years on from my eighteenth birthday, I still knew how to party. I was disappointed not to be in the bar with everyone else, but I rationalised it. After a day of travelling, I had still managed to sit through a meal *and* talk afterwards. There are only so many miracles you can squeeze into one day. I changed into my pyjamas and snuggled into bed.

At eleven o'clock, I was about to fall asleep when I started feeling itchy. My body had broken out in spots. It was just an intolerance reaction – from something I had eaten, probably. So, I slathered on my antihistamine cream and went back to bed.

But I couldn't sleep. Without warning, I began to shake and sob uncontrollably. Before setting off for Ireland, I had imagined this trip as a way to escape the EBV, yet instead it had come over with me on the ferry. Outside my room, I could hear the hum of conversation from the people still up and enjoying their lives. I should have been with them, not in bed with a fever and a swollen throat and a torso covered in hives.

It was all too much. I was *sick* of this illness. I'd had worse glandular fever episodes over the years, just as I'd had worse intolerance reactions. But the contrast between my circumstances and those of my relatives in the bar was soul-destroying. Here I was among family, yet I felt like an outsider. I started crying so hard it felt like I was choking. I must have been storing up all the anger and resentment and grief, but that night it came breaking over me in a great wave.

When I phoned Mum, she struggled to decipher my words through the sobs.

'Hang on, love,' she said. 'I'm just getting ready for bed. I'll come down to you.'

Soon there was a tentative knock at my door.

'Oh, I've got the right room this time,' said Mum, barging in in her satin nightdress. 'I tried the room across the way first. I stood there whispering, "It's me, love!" and this middle-aged man opened the door.'

I wish I'd been there to see it. The way I felt at that moment, I could have done with a laugh. 'Couldn't you have put on a dressing gown?' I said.

'Didn't bring one. So, what's up?'

I lifted my pyjama top and showed her the mass of spots.

'Are you up to date with your antihistamines?' she asked.

I nodded.

'Were you sick? Diarrhoea?'

I shook my head.

'Not too bad, then,' she said. And it was true. The spots were already fading, so there was nothing to worry about. But the intolerance reaction had been the final straw.

'I can't take this any more,' I said.

Mum wanted to know what had brought this on. When I explained my thoughts to her she said, 'How long have you felt this way?'

I shrugged. I hadn't really known that I *was* feeling that way until then.

Mum lay down on the bed. 'If it helps, people have been gushing about you tonight.'

'I find that hard to believe.'

'It's true. I didn't know you'd gone to bed. I was looking everywhere for you to see how you were. I finally asked Angela if she'd seen you.'

'Which one is she?'

'First cousin.'

'Small and blond?'

'No, that's Emer. Tall and brunette. So, I said to her, "Have you seen my daughter?" And she said, "Which one's your daughter?" When I described you to her, she said, "Oh, you mean the pretty one?"'

I blinked. 'You must have thought she'd got the wrong person.'

'I did at first.'

'Cheers.'

'Well, these days I can only see how dreadful you look.'

'Really not helping, Mum.'

Mum plumped up a pillow and put it behind her neck. 'Anyway, I described what you were wearing, and she *did* mean you! Then I talked to a few of your aunts and uncles, and they all said how elegant you are.'

I laughed.

'And how clever, too,' Mum added. 'I told them you were even sharper without the brain fog.'

Lying there in her nighty and chattering away, she looked like such a proud mother. I was so touched it made me teary again.

'That was supposed to help you,' she said.

But it didn't help. I mean, I liked the sound of this smart, pretty woman, and I'd have loved to have been her. But I wasn't. I was a pale, disabled wreck, and I hated that people didn't recognise the illness. It felt like I was living a lie. More crying and nose-running followed. 'They should see me now,' I said.

'Would you rather they didn't see your good qualities?' asked Mum.

'No,' I said. 'I just want them to understand my illness.'

*

Next thing I knew, it was morning. Mum was under the duvet next to me, her eyes wide open.

'Did I sleep?' I asked.

'A little.'

'Did *you* sleep?'

'Not really.'

While Mum sneaked back to her own room, I had a shower and prepared to face the world. Mum suggested we take a walk into town with my brother and his partner to see what Kilkenny had to offer. I vaguely remember passing an art gallery, some boutiques, an ice cream parlour, but I was still in an emotional daze. At one stage, we were crossing a bridge when a family of ducks came swimming along the river below us. I love ducks. The sight of them lifted my spirits at a time when everything else seemed bleak. But my head was obviously still in the wrong gear, because I signalled to the others and shouted, 'Look at the dicks!'

As luck would have it, a group of nuns was walking past at that moment. They stopped and stared at me. Outside the nearby shops, tourists turned to see where I was pointing.

Everyone burst out laughing. For a second, I didn't know what I'd done wrong. I had to really *think* about what I had said.

'I meant ducks,' I explained sheepishly, and the nuns resumed their strolls with smirks on their faces.

I wasn't aware of this at the time, but I was suffering with hypothyroidism on that trip. On my return home, my blood tests confirmed this, and I wondered if my meltdown and muddled words had been exacerbated by low thyroxine levels.

Whether hypothyroidism played a part or not, Kilkenny was a huge turning point for me. For a while there, I had lost all faith in my body and my future. But the fact that I bounced back so swiftly gave me huge self-confidence. I realised I had to find a way to live with my illness because I might have to battle it forever. Falling ill is a terrifying thing for people who are used to being in control, and I'd spent the last six years clinging on to a dream that was becoming more distant by the day. I had to find a way to accept what had happened and follow where my body led. There's a huge difference between giving up and letting go.

As a result of all this, Kilkenny feels like a special, almost spiritual, city to me. My family just remembers it as the place where I yelled 'dicks'.

*

Back in Durham, I spent months recovering in bed. It was clear I wouldn't be well enough to start my part-time degree in September, but Jon and I decided to move to Leeds regardless. Jon said I could reapply for the course the following year, and I said, 'Yeah, maybe.' But deep down I knew it was the end of my fledgling science career. There was only so long I could spend chasing rainbows.

I passed my days alone in my dressing gown, lost and demoralised. Then one day the doorbell rang, and I opened it to find a smiling young man carrying a black-bound Bible.

'Are you a Jehovah's Witness?' I asked. 'Because if so, you're wasting your time with me, I'm afraid.'

His smile broke into an appreciative laugh. 'Not a Jehovah's witness, no. But I am a… Bible student.'

Tomayto, tomahto. 'From where?'

'From down the bank.' Then, before I could make my excuses, he added, 'I won't keep you long, but there's a passage I want to read to you.'

There was something about him. A certain… aura. I was transfixed. He opened his Bible and said, 'I'm going to read to you from Revelations. You don't have to believe everything in that book, because it talks about dragons and other weird creatures you wouldn't like.' When he said the bit about dragons, he flapped his arms as if to simulate their flight. I found myself giggling. 'But there's one section you need to hear.'

He cleared his throat, then began reading something about how as long as I had hope, God's angels would wipe the tears from my eyes. It was the most beautiful passage from the Bible I'd ever heard. While the stranger read, he looked up from time to time as if to assure himself I hadn't shut the door on him.

Then, when his reading was finished, he nodded and turned away. No goodbye, no parting words of wisdom.

Bemused, I closed the door.

My head was spinning. I was thinking about Bible Man's words and how relevant they were to my life. I also wondered whether he was genuinely a stranger, or if he'd somehow known my story before he knocked.

I opened the door to ask him, but he was nowhere to be seen. A fast walker, obviously, or maybe he'd called on one of the neighbours. A part of me wanted to go after him – dressing gown, slippers, and all. It might earn me some odd looks, but at least that way I'd get answers.

Then I realised I didn't care about an explanation. All that mattered was that, by some weird twist of fortune, Bible Man's reading had been exactly what I needed to hear. I've heard it said that to be happy in life you need three things: something to do, someone to love, and something to hope for.

Bible Man had given me my hope back.

Chapter 11

The following weekend, there was an interesting letter in the alternative health section of *The Sunday Times*. Someone had written in to ask the resident nutritional therapist if there were any good remedies for glandular fever. The reply suggested elderberry extract and recommended a particular brand.

'You should try that,' said my mum, passing the newspaper to me.

I looked it up on the internet. It definitely had some good research behind it.[3] Feeling hopeful, I phoned all the health-food shops in my area, but none sold elderberry extract. I looked up the website of the manufacturer. There was a stockist in London.

Next morning, I phoned Jon at work. 'Is your flat near Wandsworth?' I asked.

---

3   Elderberry flavonoids contain substances that inhibit neuraminidase, a chemical that EBV (and other viruses) has on its surface. EBV uses neuraminidase to get inside your cells, and to release its progeny viruses into your bloodstream. I believed I had found my perfect antiviral: a natural neuraminidase inhibitor 'with no side effects'. However, I later read that elderberry may also make the immune system more active generally, so it is not recommended if you have an autoimmune disease. I'm not sure I would have risked trying elderberry if I had been aware of this. But I'm so glad now that I did.

'No.'

'What about your office?'

He laughed. 'Do you have any geographical knowledge of London at all? What's in Wandsworth, anyway?'

So, I told him about the health-food store, and he said he would see what he could do. But as he was negotiating a multimillion-pound contract at that moment, it might have to wait.

Honestly, priorities.

That Friday evening Jon came up to Durham and, slapping his briefcase onto the kitchen table, said, 'I've got a present for you.'

My mind raced. He often picked up little things for me like jewellery or lingerie. Things that showed me he considered me attractive and not just ill. But this time I saw not a prettily wrapped parcel but three green jars with golden lids.

'You got my elderberry!' I said, grabbing him around the neck and kissing him. 'You're amazing.'

'And *you're* easily pleased. Most girls want diamonds.'

I took the maximum dose of the capsules all weekend. At first I didn't feel any effect. But by Tuesday, when my health would normally be at its worst following a weekend with Jon, my face was no rounder and my brain fog no worse. By the time the jar was finished, my head felt clearer and I even had some colour in my cheeks. Before starting the second jar, I took a break from the pills to see if my body could retain this level of health on its own.

It couldn't. After a few days off the capsules, I started sliding back down the glandular fever slope.

*

Lying under my duvet one day, I wondered if I would ever find fulfilment. I had never been one of those girls who longed for a husband and babies. My soul was only satisfied when my head was buzzing. If I couldn't be a scientist, I needed to find another way to let my brain go mad with ideas. Without that, I would wilt.

I thought about the other things I was interested in apart from science, and eventually I settled on nutrition. The more I read about the subject, the more I realised how much there was for me to learn. And taking elderberry had shown me the improvements it could bring about. Maybe I could make other people better from what I learnt too?

I decided to look into becoming a nutritional practitioner. There were surprisingly few colleges in the country that offered accredited nutrition diplomas, and none of them was close to Durham. But there was one I liked the look of that operated via distance learning. It was a three-year course, yet the college gave people up to five years to complete it, and when I called them up to explain my condition, I was assured that if I relapsed I would be given extra time on top of that. I signed up straight away.

When the first module dropped onto my doormat, I eagerly ripped open the jiffy bag and got started. The course provided everything that appeals to my nerdish side – essay writing, drawing diagrams and explaining molecular reactions. But I was frustrated by how little I could do before my EBV called time. Just twenty or thirty minutes of studying was enough to trigger my brain fog. If I tried to push through it, I would be ill for the next month with swollen glands and a high temperature.

My mum bought me some books to help my studies,

including one called *Friendly Food*. It explained that environmental triggers, such as a bout of glandular fever, can change your sensitivity to certain food chemicals. After a couple of months of recording everything I ate, it became apparent that a few of my symptoms, like the red lines and the hives on my torso, were being brought on or exacerbated by salicylates and amines – chemicals found at high levels in foods such as tomatoes, pineapples, cured meats and stock cubes (if you want to know more, there are lists readily available online). So, I cut down on the offending foods, and my flare-ups became a rarity rather than the norm.

With my health thus slightly improved, I was able to spend more time on my nutrition course. I still had to push myself to get my half-hours of study completed, but I learnt to stop when my body told me to do so. I was living permanently on the cliff edge of a glandular fever relapse. Still, that was better than falling off it.

*

Around this time, Jon's workload was particularly heavy, and as I alternated between studying and relapsing, he was working through the nights and at weekends. His health began to suffer. He came down with shingles, then developed chest pains. One Friday night, he arrived in Durham looking gaunt and grey-skinned.

My mum eagerly got out her stethoscope and pressed it to his chest. 'Gosh,' she said. 'I haven't heard one of those since I was in med school.'

'A heart?' I asked.

'A friction rub. It's pericarditis. Have a listen.'

'No, you're alright,' I said. But it was no good. I had a stethoscope shoved in my ears anyway and was told to listen for the 'click' with each beat.

Pericarditis is inflammation of the heart lining caused, in Jon's case, by an underlying viral infection. When Mum's diagnosis was later confirmed by a cardiologist in London, Jon was signed off work. I decided to go and stay with him. I had now found an online supplier of elderberry extract and was taking it continually so, for once, I felt well enough to travel. I thought we could convalesce together.

Towards the end of my stay, Jon had a check-up with his GP. I went to the appointment with him. The inflammation around his heart was receding, and his blood tests showed the virus was on its way out. But Jon said he felt just as ill.

'That's because you now have Post-Viral Fatigue Syndrome,' said the doctor.

At first I thought I must have misheard. I was stunned that Jon could be labelled with that term so readily. After all, he still had residual symptoms of pericarditis and shingles. So why couldn't the GP just say it would take Jon a while longer to regain full health? Why had he slapped a frightening new diagnosis on him?

His words struck a nerve. I myself had been labelled with Post-Viral Fatigue Syndrome a hundred times, and I didn't find the term helpful because there was nothing 'post' about my virus – the EBV remained active in my system. And now the same diagnosis was being given to Jon. How could my illness be compared to his? How could people with relapsing conditions like mine be grouped together with people who simply took longer than 'normal' to recover from their illnesses? It wasn't helpful to either group of patients. More importantly, how would researchers ever get to the bottom of PVFS/ME/CFS if people were so casually diagnosed with it?

In the black cab on the way back to Jon's flat, these thoughts raced through my mind. Jon shuffled across the leather seat and wrapped his arms around me.

'There you go again with your furrowed brow.' He stroked my forehead, as if to iron out the creases. 'Do you think you could manage a short break away with me? I'm not allowed to fly while I've got pericarditis, so it would have to be somewhere close.'

And that is how, a few years after our holiday to Barcelona, our trip to Bordeaux came about.

*

'The chest pains have returned,' said Jon as he parked the car on the ferry to Caen. 'Shall we find somewhere to rest?'

At the customer services desk, we tried to get a cabin, only to find they had all been pre-booked. So, we wandered around the decks looking for somewhere to flop and eventually discovered a lounge with reclining seats.

'Strange how you really need to lie down flat when you're feeling ill,' said Jon. 'A reclining chair just isn't *proper* rest, is it?'

He would say things like that during his illness – things that I think every day of my life, and that I wish people would instinctively grasp. It helped, having Jon's understanding of what it was like to be ill long-term: the determination to keep things outwardly normal versus the need to constantly lie down.

By the time we reached our apartment in Bordeaux, Jon looked grey again, and I was a bit yellow. A perfect match to the external colour scheme of the apartment blocks. 'How are we going to get better?' Jon asked, as we stared out across our balcony into the coniferous forest.

'Chicken soup!' I said. Because it's full of antivirals and anti-inflammatories and… OK, I'll stop now.

We popped to the local shop and bought the ingredients. But after five minutes battling with a chicken carcass, Jon conceded defeat and slumped down in a chair in the living area. I carried on chopping for a little longer, then felt my face start to swell up. Heavy eyed, I put down my knife and joined Jon on the sofa.

'How do you live like this?' he asked.

'Got no choice, babe. Gotta look towards the future. I'm not going to be ill forever, you know.'

'I hope not. I hope we both recover.'

'*We*? You'll be fine in a month or two. And I'll be OK… eventually.' I glanced back into the kitchen. 'Maybe the soup was a bit ambitious. Maybe we should stick to wine tasting.'

Jon didn't need convincing. The next day, we drove out into the countryside with a pile of wine guides, tracking down vineyards that were open to the public. The French wine makers warmed to this young, pale, English couple, and kept taking us into their living rooms to show us pictures of their ancestors while topping up our glasses.

Jon's chest pains began to abate, and he regained some colour. When it was time to go back to the UK, I knew he at least was on the road to recovery. I, on the other hand, took months to pull out of my ensuing relapse. Jon said that he would never forget what it was like having a long-term illness, especially one which, rightly or wrongly, had been labelled as Post-Viral Fatigue Syndrome. But life moves on for the healthy, and a year or so later he admitted that not only did he have no memory of being so ill, but he had also forgotten saying those words to me as well!

Perhaps I should marvel at the resilience of the human body and its mind. And perhaps that should give hope to some of the readers of this book. But as thrilled as I was for Jon, it also made me feel that once again I was alone with my health battles, and alone with the emotions that went with them.

*

As another year of illness passed, I decided I had to get on with the next chapter of my life as best I could. Jon suggested that we meet in Leeds whenever health permitted. He was due to start work there the following January, so we needed to find somewhere to live. New year, new start.

Same old illness.

Those weekend breaks to Leeds were some of the happiest moments of my life. After five years of long-distance dating, Jon and I were choosing where to set up home. It was hard knowing what would suit our lifestyle when we didn't know what sort of life my health would permit. So, we viewed everything from trendy apartments in the centre of town to draughty three-storey houses further out. At the end, when we stopped for lunch at a pub, I looked at the pool table longingly – not because I wanted to play, but because I wished I could stretch out on it to recover.

Back in Durham, Mum used my remaining time at home to get things fixed around the house. One morning, as I tucked into yet another jar of elderberry, she asked if I could let in a plumber the following day. I said it would be fine, but my eyes must have given me away because she asked me what was so taxing about unlocking a door for a workman.

I explained that it wasn't just putting a key in a lock and turning it. Not only would I need to get washed and dressed, but I'd also have to explain to the guy what needed doing, because he wouldn't have been listening when Mum gave instructions. Then I would be forced to listen while he showed off about how bad the last workman was, and what he'd do to fix his mistakes. And as I made him his tenth cup of coffee or hunted out our dustpan and brush…well, there went another chunk of health.

Silence. Mum looked devastated. She said she would never let a workman near the house again until I left home. Guilt had sunk its claws into her, and she started asking about other things that affected my health. For example, when she and Dad held a dinner party, and they asked me to 'rustle up' a pavlova, did that make me worse too?

'Yes,' I said. 'But I want to do these things for you.'

'You are never to cook for us again!' she declared.

We squared up to each other like gunslingers in a Western.

'Yes, I am. Starting with when your friends come over next week.'

'No,' she said. 'I'm going to buy a dessert from Marks and Spencer.'

'Well, it'll be going straight in the freezer, then. Because by the time you come back from the shops, *my* dessert will already be prepared.'

'I'd refuse to eat it on principle.'

'You hate waste.'

'I'd give it away, then!'

'Good! Then at least someone will benefit from my otherwise pointless existence.'

We stared at each other for a few seconds. Then Mum reached over and gave me a hug. I cried into her shoulder, momentarily lost for words.

Eventually I said, 'I hope your top isn't dry-clean only.'

Mum smiled. 'I know you think you're a burden, but you're not. You're a joy. And if you really want to help me, then do everything you can to get better. That means no more pavlovas.'

I reluctantly nodded, but I couldn't shake off the feeling I was useless. I was a doer in life. And if I couldn't even do my share about the house, what sort of partner was I going to be? I wasn't prepared to be one of those princess-like women who make their men dance around doing everything for them.

No way.

*

It was early February, and Jon was in Durham for the weekend. On Sunday, he suggested we go for a drink at Lumley Castle – a historic hotel in nearby Chester-le-Street. I took some convincing. It was just a couple of hours before Jon was due to catch a train back to London, but he was clearly keen to end his stay on a high, so I let myself be persuaded.

At that time, Shakira was storming the charts with her song, 'Whenever, Wherever'. So as Jon and I sped down the motorway, I turned up the radio and sang along to the chorus. I looked at Jon, sad at the thought of him leaving so soon, and said, 'You know the lyrics are true, don't you? That we're meant to be together.'

He laughed but didn't answer. Instead, he took his hand off the gear stick and gave mine a squeeze.

I was still humming as we strolled hand in hand through the castle courtyards to the library bar with its roaring fires and brooding portraits. While Jon went to order the drinks, I collapsed onto a padded velvet seat and started to read the spines of some of the antique books in the bookcases surrounding me. So many of them were medical in nature; it felt like there was no escape from illness.

'Penny for them?' asked Jon as he put my pot of tea down on the table. 'I leave you singing along to Shakira and return to find The Furrowed Brow.'

'Just goes to show, you should never leave me,' I joked.

'You know I won't.'

He sat beside me, and we talked about all the great weekends we had had together during our five years of dating. We had visited castles in North Yorkshire, beaches in County Durham, forts along Hadrian's Wall… But Jon hardly remembered these stunning locations. For him, it was never about where we were, but how we felt. We were soon chatting about what our future would be like when I was better.

'I think I might want two kids, two guinea pigs, and a dog,' I said.

'You can't have just one dog,' replied Jon. 'It'll get lonely.'

'It can play with the kids.'

'It's not the same. It needs another dog friend.'

'Fine. Two of everything, then.' It never crossed my mind that I might not be well enough to look after six dependents.

We left the bar, smiling. Then Jon suggested a circuit around the castle before going home.

'Sorry, I can't,' I said. 'It's been a long weekend, and I'm blobbing up.'

'Just one lap.'

I was taken aback. Normally Jon was the one making me rest, but instead I found him dragging me around to the side of the castle. We halted beneath two huge flags hanging from the main towers. There was no noise apart from the caw of a crow on the battlements. Jon was looking serious.

'Are you alright?' I asked.

'Yes,' he said. But he didn't look it. Perhaps a kiss would lift his mood, two to be safe.

Still the earnest expression.

I was stumped. We had had such a relaxed time in the bar, so what had brought on this solemn expression? I was still trying to work it out when a gust of wind set the flags above us flapping, and Jon took a breath, looked at me, and said, 'Lily, will you marry me?'

Chapter 12

'Is this for real?' I asked Jon.

'Because the old fool-your-ill-girlfriend-with-a-fake-proposal trick is such a classic,' he replied, deadpan.

'No, it's just… I wasn't expecting it. But yes! Of course!'

Jon hugged me before raising an eyebrow and saying, 'Oh, so you do like some surprises, then?'

'I can't believe you've got to go back to London now. Tell me you don't have to go.'

'I don't have to go.'

'What?'

'I've taken tomorrow off. I thought maybe we could go ring shopping. In fact, while we're here, I thought we could book Lumley Castle for our wedding reception next year. What do you think?'

'I think I like your style.'

Back at home, I rushed in to share the news with my parents. Soon Dad was chilling the champagne, and just for a few minutes I felt like a newly engaged girl should feel: exhilarated and whole. But the more we celebrated, the sicker I became. My immune system wouldn't even let me enjoy this moment without a 'but'.

I called Caja to tell her the news and ask her to be a bridesmaid.

'Didn't I tell you that you two would end up married?' she squealed. 'Do you remember that night in the Italian restaurant in Cambridge? I knew you'd met Mr Right, didn't I?'

'You did,' I said. I had known it too, and the memory of that determined student desperately trying to quash her feelings made me smile. It felt like a lifetime ago.

'What colour will I be wearing?' asked Caja.

'Colour? You do know I only got engaged today, don't you?'

There was a pause. 'You mean you haven't been planning your wedding since you were a little girl?'

'No.'

'Well, what have you been daydreaming about all these years?'

'My Nobel Prize.'

She laughed.

The celebrations commenced. People descended on the house with cards and gifts. It was so kind, so heartfelt, so… exhausting. The ring shopping with Jon had already tipped me into a relapse, but I didn't have the heart to turn anyone away.

Next came the wedding planning. It was difficult spacing out all the things that had to be done, from meeting with the priest to discuss the service, to travelling to a wedding fair, to sorting out cars. I sank further and further into illness. That's one of the worst aspects of my condition: it can make even the most treasured events in life seem hard.

To make matters worse, around this time I had to attend

a number of lecture days on my nutritional practitioner's course. They were held in hotels at Manchester airport. I could take my pick from the dates available, but without a working crystal ball I had no way of knowing when I would be well enough to travel. All too often, when the day came around, I found myself sweating in bed instead of sitting at a lecture.

When I *was* able to attend course days, my parents had to drive me there and back. Those lectures took a heavy toll on my health, but I always came away feeling happier because I was doing something I loved.

It was good for me to mix with strangers again too. Yet, it was difficult knowing how much to tell them about my illness. When you meet someone for the first time, the obvious questions they ask are, 'What do you do for a living?' and, 'If you don't work, what do you do all day?' I had to either skirt around the issue or fess up that I was disabled.

Coming clean was harder than you might expect. If I told people what my life was like, they often didn't understand or, worse, seemed not to believe me. On the few occasions that I did see a flicker of comprehension – the shock, the pity – their response highlighted how tragic they thought my circumstances were.

*

December was fast approaching. I know Christmas is a magical time for most, but all I wanted from Santa each year was to emerge from the season unscathed. There were so many things to do, and so little health with which to do them. It started with writing Christmas cards to all the people I had been neglecting. I would begin in November, determined to write one a day so I finished in time, only for my ill health to disrupt proceedings and leave me scribbling them all at the last minute.

Mum begged me not to bother, but I felt that since I'd been too ill to speak to these people for an entire year, the least I could do was show them I was thinking of them at Christmas. In reality, I thought of them daily. It annoyed me that I had been cut off from friends and relatives. But judging by things that some have told me, it annoyed them even more.

Then there was the present buying. One year I was so ill from October to Christmas, my mum had to buy my presents for me from a list I had painstakingly compiled. When a relative asked me where their gift was from, I was embarrassed to admit I didn't know. Eventually, they found the item in Asda at a much cheaper price, and the episode made them think I hadn't put in any effort at all. Awkward.

Each Christmas morning, the banging and crashing in the kitchen always woke me at seven. I would appear in my fluffy slippers and offer to help Dad with the food.

'No, it's all under control,' he'd assure me as he sawed off the turkey's legs to make it fit in the oven. Then he would offer me bubbly, and I'd say something like, 'But it's only seven in the morning!' before letting him convince me to have a glass on the pretence it might relieve the brain fog.

Later, as I stood in church singing 'Hark! The Herald Angels Sing' while toddlers played in the pews with their new toys, I would find myself swaying on my feet. And not to the music, either. Jon says that most time at Catholic Mass is spent standing up, sitting down and kneeling, and I soon came to realise he was right. Ten minutes into every service, I would desperately need a lie-down to help me recover from the aerobics.

By Boxing Day, I was always ill with a capital 'I'. The day after that, Jon and I would meet up with his family in Nottingham. The journey and the socialising were the final nail in my health's coffin. While at home, I could rest in bed whenever I needed to. But in the company of other people, I rarely had the courage to steal away when I was flagging. I didn't have the health to be more involved, or the words to explain my illness properly. And because of this, Jon's relatives couldn't realise how much my condition inhibited me.

*

That year, my Christmas relapse only lasted one month instead of the usual three. By the start of February, I was able to catch a train to begin my new life with Jon in Leeds. When we think back to our time there, we agree it was bittersweet. The first morning when I woke up beside Jon, the sun's rays were filtering through the hideous floral curtains of our rented apartment. I actually thought (feel free to vomit), *that's like my hope filtering through my illness*. I wrote in my diary that morning that I knew I was going to get better.

Every weekend we looked for wedding dresses and rings together. One Saturday, Jon's Y chromosomes couldn't take any more 'girly' shops, so he asked if he could redress his hormonal balance by looking at computer games in WHSmith. As we climbed the stairs to the upper floor, I realised I was too ill to reach the top. So, I sat down on the steps, head clouding over, and told Jon I would wait for him there.

He had only been gone a few minutes when three generations of Yorkshire women came strutting down the stairs with overflowing carrier bags. The grandma – a burly, steel-haired woman in a checked coat – stopped and stared at me.

'You alright, pet?' she asked.

'Fine, thanks.'

'No, you're not. You're as white as milk.' She lowered herself onto the stained, green fluff of my stair. 'Are you on your own?'

'Mam, come on!' yelled her daughter from the bottom of the steps.

'No,' I told the grandma. 'My fiancé is upstairs. He'll be down in a minute.'

'Mam!'

'Shurrup! Can't you see the poor lass is about to faint?'

Jon must have heard the commotion because at that moment he came striding down the stairs. 'What's going on?' He smiled at the old woman.

She glared back at him. 'Right you are,' she said to me, then pushed herself upright. 'You look after her properly,' she told Jon, a little too brusquely.

I had to look away to stop myself laughing.

I have always remembered this incident because of that gruff lady's compassion. There were times in life when friends who perhaps should have been there for me barely acknowledged I was ill. Yet this stranger cared enough that she refused to leave until Jon returned. It proved to me that there were thoughtful people out there who didn't require a medical diagnosis to show concern for someone who just appeared pale.

'Do I really look that dreadful?' I asked Jon when we were alone.

'No worse than normal,' he said. I shot him a death stare, and he laughed. 'I mean, you do look ill, but you're still gorgeous. So, more ring shopping? Or have you reached your limit?'

'Passed it a long time ago. Can we go home?'

Later that day, while resting in bed, I drifted off into a nightmare where my mum took me to New York to find a ring I liked. The dream ended with me picking up a chest infection on the plane back and being too ill to attend my own wedding.

*

As well as planning a wedding, Jon and I were now looking for a house to buy. So, in between the dress and the ring shopping, we spent our time traipsing around people's homes, scratching for positive things to say. The owners would proudly point out the underfloor heating, the handcrafted banisters, the French doors opening onto the garden. But the thing that drew my eye most was always the beds. I yearned to lie down and heal.

People said to us, why did we need to live in a family house when there was just the two of us? Half of them assumed we were trying to keep up with the Joneses; the other half wondered if I was pregnant. What nobody seemed to appreciate was that home was where I spent ninety-nine per cent of my life. It had to be the loveliest, most spacious place we could afford so that it felt like my refuge and not my prison. And I wanted a garden so that on those days when I was too ill to get dressed, I could at least stagger outside in my dressing gown to get some fresh air.

We finally settled on a modern house in a cul-de-sac, and the sale went through in July – one month before we were due to get married. While I was recovering from the move, three significant things happened: I turned twenty-six, I got my first wrinkle, and I came down with a flu-like bug that sent my temperature into orbit. Unable even to answer the phone, I'd receive texts from friends asking me when my final dress fitting was, or if Jon and I were having dance lessons for our first dance.

Dancing? I was barely able to text back. In the end, my family and bridesmaids stepped into the breach. My mum was left to handle the seating plan and the guests' accommodation, not to mention the thousand-and-one things that typically go wrong in the lead up to a wedding.

I didn't have a hen do. My bridesmaids suggested that we go to a health farm for a weekend and lounge about in the jacuzzi. I felt dreadful when I had to turn them down. The packing, the talking, and the dressing up for meals would have triggered a relapse when I could least afford it. If I was going to make it to the church at all, I needed my own home and no interruptions.

When my wedding day came around, the service was in the afternoon so I had the whole morning to get ready. I showered, then had a lie-down. I got my hair done, then had a lie-down. I did my make-up, then ran a half-marathon.

Only kidding.

None of my guests will have realised the lengths I went

to just to get to the church. Most brides want the perfect day, but I settled for being able to walk down the aisle unaided. In the car on the way, I tried to keep quiet in order to conserve health. But my dad mistook my silence for anxiety and started telling bad jokes to ease my 'nerves'. In the end I had to chat to him to ensure he didn't resort to his customary singing.

On the way into the church, I was stopped by the photographer for the obligatory father-and-bride shots. Under my breath, I prayed I wasn't looking half as bad as I felt, because no bride wants a football-head in the photos. Inside, when I saw Jon in front of the altar, smiling back at me, I thought of the guy who had flashed me that same smile across the dance floor at Cambridge seven years ago. And now here we were – it was perfect.

Well, *nearly* perfect.

Because as my face swelled up across the day, I was forced to take frequent rests in a room adjacent to the banqueting suite. The 'hole' inside me that I'd first acknowledged in Malta was still present. I felt like I was merely playing the role of the happy bride, and not even Jon's reassuring hand squeezes could dispel that thought. To those around me, I must have seemed like any other newlywed, smiling and air-kissing. But inside I was battling through my sludgy brain and trying to ignore the pains in my joints. I didn't want to be *acting* good health; I wanted to *be* well.

Jon gets a little despondent when we talk about that day. He says it was the best moment of his life, but I can't honestly say it was mine. I prefer to remember the days he and I shared that weren't affected by my condition. Happiness means something different when you're constantly fighting illness. For me, true contentment can only be found on the days that I escape the EBV's shadow.

One of those times came on honeymoon when Jon and I were driving down a leafy Provencal avenue. The fragrance of lavender was in the air, and I experienced a sense of joy and release that I hadn't felt since my Cambridge days. I laughed, and when Jon asked why, I said, 'Because the hole just disappeared!'

He didn't understand, so he pulled over to the side of the road and made me explain. I told him about my sense of loss over missing out on so much in life. I explained about my uncertainty over what future my health would allow, and how my concerns had all disappeared briefly. They returned soon enough, but the fact that they had gone away at all made me confident that one day neither my illness nor my lack of a career would matter to me any more. I would find fulfilment.

Chapter 13

Back home in Leeds, Jon attempted to carry me over the threshold, but my gangly legs crashed against the door frame.

'Hang on, let's try something else,' he said, putting me down. Suddenly I was hauled into a fireman's lift and lowered onto the carpet on the other side. 'Welcome home, Mrs Whelan.'

I had returned from my honeymoon healthier than I had left, but the enormity of what awaited me was clear when I scanned the house. There were boxes from the move to be unpacked, pictures to be hung, cleaning to be tackled—

'Stop it!' said Jon, seeing my expression. 'It's going to be fine.'

He was probably right. What was the hurry? It didn't matter if it took us six months to make the house presentable. Like everything else in my life, housework could only be tackled in bitesize portions so as not to trigger a glandular fever relapse.

As it turned out, the travelling triggered a relapse anyway, and it took me the rest of the year to recover. In December, one of Jon's work colleagues invited us to a New Year's Eve party, but I was in no fit state to go. Instead, in the run-up to midnight, Jon and I snuggled up on the sofa and watched an episode of *The Office*. As I laughed along, I glanced out of the bay window into the clear black night and saw it was snowing. Dragging Jon over to the window, I said, 'Isn't it beautiful!' And probably because he'd been drinking, he agreed.

Many years later, a friend of Jon asked him what his best New Year's Eve was. I was theoretically out of earshot, so I waited with bated breath to hear what amazing event with which healthy former girlfriend he would choose. Instead, he said, 'My first New Year's Eve in Leeds with Lily.' He didn't mention how ill I had been. Possibly, he didn't even remember.

Uplifted, I told myself off for thinking that my illness ruined everything. It *changed* everything, yes. It made our life together evolve in a way we hadn't anticipated. But whatever else happened, I knew we would always find happiness together.

*

Six months later, I was seeing to a workman who was laying laminate flooring in the spare bedroom. He was a lovely person, polite and genuine. I asked him how long he'd been fitting floors, and he told me this wasn't his usual line of work. He had been forced to leave his office job due to ill health. The floor-laying was a way to bring in money while he recovered.

As he worked, he told me about his illness – a kidney disease that had led to him needing steroids.

I said, 'Are you sticking to the diet they gave you?'

'What diet?'

I covered my surprise. 'Didn't the doctor give you a diet sheet for your condition?'

'No.'

'But he must have referred you to a dietician?'

'No, there was no talk of food at all,' the workman replied, head down as he locked two boards together.

'If you like, I could tell you what you should be eating.'

He paused and looked at me. 'That would be great.'

As I headed upstairs to consult my notes, my thoughts were abuzz with excitement.

From implementing all I had learnt from my nutrition books, papers and modules, I had succeeded in improving my condition – albeit marginally. Now I had the chance to do the same for someone else.

Two sides of A4 later, I was finished. As the workman was packing up his tools, I handed him the paper. He asked how much I wanted.

'How much what?' I asked.

'How much money.'

'I don't want to be paid. I just want you to follow the diet so you get better.'

'Why?'

'Sorry?'

'You don't know me. Why would you care?'

It seemed a strange thing to ask. A better question would be, why *wouldn't* I care? I thought about mentioning my own illness. When you struggle every day, you develop a passion to relieve the suffering of others. That sounded a bit melodramatic, though, so I shrugged and changed the subject.

Later, I found out through an alternative therapist we shared that the workman was sticking to his diet and feeling the benefits. The news ignited something within me. If I could just get better, I could start making a difference to my small corner of the world.

*

Jon and I had been living in our new house in Leeds for almost a year before we acquainted ourselves with our neighbours. At a barbeque one weekend, they admitted to having considered us 'mysterious'. Each day, Jon left early in the morning and arrived back late at night. And then there was me, always wearing a dressing gown and rarely leaving the house. When I told them our story, they probably wished they hadn't asked. Reality rarely lives up to the mystery. I should have told them we were spies instead.

Unfortunately, as soon as we'd got to know our neighbours, it was time to say goodbye. Jon wasn't enjoying his new job, and since moving to Leeds, my health had taken a nosedive. I won't bore you with the ins and outs of my daily routine. But in short, when I wasn't dragging myself to the surgery or the hospital, I was trying and failing to run the house by myself. With Jon's long working hours, he could never be around to help me.

One Saturday afternoon, he asked me what I thought about moving back to Durham. I had mixed emotions. I associated Leeds with wedding shopping and with starting a new life. Whereas Durham felt like sick land because of the years I'd spent there alone with my glandular fever. Then again, in the Northeast I would have my parents close by, not to mention the immunology department at the RVI in Newcastle. Whatever memories Durham might hold, going back there was the right move for my recovery.

Once Jon handed in his notice, everything happened quickly. The day the 'For Sale' board was hammered into our front lawn, a man came round for a viewing and offered us the asking price. With no time to find a house in Durham, we put our belongings into storage and moved in with my parents.

I remember my first appointment back with Dr Spickett in Newcastle. When I told him I wasn't well enough to live independently, he responded, 'Of course you are!' and his comment made my heart sink. I knew he was just trying to bolster my self-belief. My friends and family would often tell me what they thought I wanted to hear, but sometimes their positivity made it seem like they didn't understand how incapacitated I was. I didn't need them to tell me what I was or wasn't capable of doing – only I knew that.

I enjoyed being back with my parents, but having had a taste of freedom, I was keen to have my own space again. Almost as keen, no doubt, as they were to see me gone. Within a few weeks, my mum was already beginning to show the strains of having to nurse her sick daughter again.

'Do you think you need a holiday?' I asked her.

There was a glimmer of amusement in her eyes. 'Trying to get the house to yourselves, are you?'

'No! I didn't mean...' Then I considered. 'Although now you mention it...'

'It's OK. Dad and I are thinking of going to France. Maybe by the time we're back, you'll have found yourselves a nice house.'

'Is that a hint?'

'Yes.'

While they were away, we found our own home, a stroll away from Jon's new office. The kitchen was crumbling and the carpets were glow-in-the-dark pink, but its spaciousness and its abundance of natural light made it the perfect place for me to convalesce. The rest was down to me and the EBV.

Chapter 14

Now that I was back in Durham, I could let the people I knew and trusted assist with the chores. A family friend came over once a week to clean and hoover, and my mum dropped by regularly to collect laundry. Our neighbours saw us passing bags full of clothing between us and asked if we did lots of shopping for each other. They were also curious as to why I spent so much of my life in my dressing gown.

They weren't the only ones puzzled about my attire. One afternoon, my mum called on me at home and looked aghast when she noticed what I was wearing.

'Dear Lord!' she cried. 'Tell me your mother-in-law doesn't see you in that dressing gown.'

'Of course not,' I replied. 'This is my scruffy-wear dressing gown. I wear my best-wear dressing gown for guests and when I go into hospital. I also have a medium-wear dressing gown for everything else.'

'You have three grades of dressing gown?' she asked, bewildered.

I nodded. 'You know, like normal people have workwear, loungewear, and formalwear.'

With the help I received from friends and family, my health

began to pick up. My glands were going down and my face was slim when Jon suggested we spend a week in Burgundy to celebrate his thirtieth birthday. On our return to Durham, Jon was unpacking a case when he turned to me and asked, 'Do you know what the best thing about the holiday was?'

Well, I like a challenge, but there were so many moments to choose from. 'Was it when the hotel receptionist upgraded us to a suite, free of charge?' I asked.

'No.'

'Was it at the wine warehouse, then, when we accidentally tagged on to the back of that tour group and ended up getting free drinks?'

Jon raised an eyebrow. '"Accidentally"? I thought it was more a case of, "the bubbly is opened, and Lily forgets her sense of morality"?'

'You forgot yours too!'

'Not sure I ever had one.'

I threw a cushion at him. 'I give up. What was the best thing about the holiday?'

He squeezed me and lifted me off the ground. 'Your health. Don't you realise? You were well for the entire trip!'

Actually, 'well' might have been overstating it. The hotel restaurant had seemed incapable of serving me a non-allergenic meal, so I had spent large parts of the trip searching for my antihistamine pills before I scratched my skin off. But otherwise, he was right. I hadn't been glandular fevery for a whole week. Consequently, we had been able to go out for part of each day. And when I looked back at the photos of the holiday, I could see my cheekbones in every one of them.

There was hope! If I continued on the path I was following, perhaps I would have more weeks like that.

*

Unfortunately, life had other ideas. Jon's sister was getting married the following month, and I was determined to attend the ceremony. I dosed myself up on paracetamol and elderberry, but the event was still more than I could cope with. The following day, I was back at home in my (scruffy-wear) dressing gown with enlarged glands and a high temperature.

Next, my dad's health took a nosedive. He'd been experiencing chest pains for a couple of months, and a scan revealed that three of his coronary arteries were ninety per cent blocked. The blockages were in such risky positions, the cardiologist called them 'widow makers'. Dad needed a triple heart bypass and was whisked off to hospital.

My mum became a wisp of her former self. She needed me, so, together with Jon, I moved back in with her. Every day, Mum and I would travel up to Newcastle to visit Dad in hospital. He was in a ward of pot-bellied, middle-aged men who had to clutch pillows to their chests so their stitched torsos wouldn't burst open when they coughed. In comparison, I looked vibrantly healthy. But in reality, my glands were ballooning with each trip to the hospital.

If I had my time again, I wouldn't do anything differently. But just before Dad was discharged from hospital, I relapsed with full-blown glandular fever. I was as ill as I had been for a couple of years. My blood tests showed I was IgM positive again, so Dr Spickett put me back on high-dose Aciclovir.

Jon drove me over to my parents' house so I could check on Dad while he recuperated. I don't know which of us looked worse: my dad lying limply in bed with his chest sewn back together, or me with my glands protruding from my neck. I reminded myself that my dad had just been sawn in half, that he had been technically dead – briefly – when his heart was stopped during his operation, and he was now on a cocktail of drugs for life, so I shouldn't expect him to look anything other than deathly.

But he still recovered faster than me.

*

While Dad was back on the golf course, I was stuck in bed with chills and swollen eyelids. Life would have been very gloomy indeed had it not been for my fantastic hubby. Jon was pleased to discover that in Durham it was possible to quit the office at five o'clock and not work at weekends. But he still found it hard leaving me when I was unwell.

One Monday morning, I sensed Jon leaning over me as I lay in bed. 'Come on,' he said. 'You can do it.'

I sighed. 'Babe, I know you mean well, but I really can't. Just go to work.'

'Not until you open your eyes.'

'Can't.'

He laughed and tugged at the duvet, and I would have laughed too if my throat didn't hurt so much. 'Fine,' he said. 'Have it your way.'

I heard his steps on the wooden floorboards as he retreated towards the door... before stopping. There was silence for a moment. Then I heard a tap, tap, tap as if he were drumming a beat on the floor.

'What are you doing?' I asked, my eyes still shut.

Jon didn't reply. The tapping continued, back and forth across the room.

It was no good, I had to look – just as Jon had intended. I heaved myself upright, prised my eyelids open, and waited for my vision to come into focus.

And there he was: Jon, of all people, dancing across the room.

'Are you… tap-dancing?' I said.

'Ah, so you *can* open your eyes,' he replied. 'And for your information, it's not tap-dancing, it's Irish dancing.'

I surveyed him more closely. 'Well, the legs could pass for Irish dancing, but I'm not sure about the jazz hands.'

'If you're going to be pedantic, I'm off to work.'

'Encore!' I said as he moved towards the stairs.

He laughed again. 'No, you had your chance.'

I sank back into the pillows, no longer caring about my eyelids, or my inability to get out of bed. Love is the best anaesthetic.

*

One day that spring, I was flaked out on the futon in the conservatory when I heard a squawk outside. I looked into the garden and saw a tiny black shape under the pergola. I slipped on my wellies and crept along the garden path for a closer look.

It was a baby crow that must have fallen out of its nest in one of the conifers at the end of the garden. It seemed happy to see me, flapping its wings and hopping over. When it opened its mouth wide, I crouched down and asked, 'Are you hungry, little one?'

It danced about, head tilted back ready to receive food.

'If I go, your mummy might come back and feed you,'

I told it. So, I retreated to the conservatory to watch what happened next.

No mother came for it. You probably think it's a bit of artistic license for me to say it looked despondent, but I swear it's the truth.

I had never seen a creature look so vulnerable. Black clouds circled as a storm blew in. The cat from across the road was prowling along the fence, planning its attack. I put my wellies back on, chased the cat away and approached the bird. Again, it opened its beak and squawked.

'Hang on,' I said.

After some time, I found it an extra thin worm and put it down on the ground. The crow pecked at the worm before looking back at me like a kid who couldn't unwrap his present.

'Sorry,' I said. Because whilst I was happy to try to feed this creature, I drew the line at regurgitation. Instead, I filled a bowl with water and put that down beside the bird in the hope it could help itself to a drink. Then I returned to the conservatory once more to recover from the exertion.

When Jon came home from work, I hurried into the hallway to greet him and tell him about the bird. I don't know what reaction I was expecting from him, but whatever it was, I didn't get it. I could see his frustration simmering. An artery pulsed in his temple.

'What?' I said. 'What's wrong with me trying to help—'

'A crow,' he cut in. 'Look at you! You're ill. You've got a temperature. Why would you want to make yourself worse?'

'It could have died.'

'Whereas your health is much less important. And where did you get the worm from, anyway? Did you get a spade and dig up the garden?'

'No, I picked it from the compost.'

'Of course you did,' he muttered. Loosening his tie, he slumped down onto one of the stairs. I squeezed in beside him.

'Don't be cross,' I said.

'I'm not cross,' he said, but the tightness in his voice suggested otherwise. 'It's your life, you can do what you want. But if you're going to make yourself sicker, at least make yourself sicker doing things for yourself. Not by helping other people. And definitely not by helping crows.'

'It was the right thing to do,' I protested. We sat in silence for a while. Then I piped up: 'Is that our annual row over? Who'd have thought it would be over a bird. We never row about things normal couples row about, do we?'

'Why, what do normal couples row about?' asked Jon.

'Oh, you know – household chores, money, sex, that sort of thing.'

'And you know this because…?'

'Because I have wasted far too much of my life reading the piles of women's magazines in hospital waiting rooms.'

Jon then pointed out that the row wasn't really about the crow, it was about me not looking after myself.

'Come on,' he said, standing up and helping me to rise too.

'Where are we going?'

'Bed.'

'Now you're talking.'

'To *rest*,' he said. But between you and me, I could tell he was tempted.

'I'll join you in a minute,' I replied. 'I've just got to do something.' I started to walk down the hallway, but he grabbed my hand and pulled me back.

'You are not going to check on that bird!' he said, laughing.

'OK. But I'm going to lie down in the guest room, not our room.' And even though he knew that was so I could look into the garden, he didn't object.

The following morning, when I went back to lie down in the spare bedroom, I heard two sets of squawks and looked out of the window to see my little crow and its mother perched on the fence. The baby gazed up and smiled at me.

OK, the smile is poetic license.

*

Jon had raised a good point, though. I *was* making myself sicker to please others. At times, like my dad's operation, that was the right thing to do. But there was a line to be drawn, and too often I was straying onto the wrong side of it.

I promised Jon I would think twice now before accepting long phone calls, or allowing guests to stay, or filling shoeboxes for charity. I felt guilty at the thought of putting myself first, but I would never get better otherwise, or have the chance to do the things I wanted. For example, I knew I would like to try for a baby at some point. But first I needed to finish my nutrition course, and to do *that* I would have to get past the dressing gown stage of my illness.

People were all too willing to share their opinions on how I should do that, but their advice was still based on false assumptions about my condition. They thought I wasn't really ill, just 'washed out' in the way that they might feel after a hard week at work. A medic once told me I'd had glandular fever for so long, I'd simply forgotten what being well felt like.

Other doctors used inaccurate petrol-tank analogies; after a virus, they would say, you have to pace yourself, because if you used up all your petrol in one go, you'd have to wait for your tank to refill.

Cue muffled scream.

Politeness and weariness stopped me from going on about it. Well, maybe I went on about it a *little*. Occasionally I would stomp around saying things like, if someone has a migraine which then becomes a less severe headache, do other people tell them that really they have no headache at all? Or that they've forgotten what no headache feels like? Of course not. So why did people insist viral infections had an expiry date, and that anyone who felt ill beyond that time must just be fatigued? It was blinkered and unfair, and one day I would make people see this.

In my calmer moments, I understood why many doctors viewed ME/CFS in this way. If they hadn't been taught about the condition at med school, they might not realise that the glandular fever virus doesn't always go properly dormant. Yet there had been research studies demonstrating that EBV could linger long past its usual time frame – I have some from as far back as the '80s and '90s, including one that concluded there was 'evidence for active EBV infection in patients with persistent, unexplained illnesses'.[a] Had articles like these hit the headlines at the time, I believe ME/CFS cases such as mine would be viewed differently. But such studies rarely made the news, unlike the prejudiced viewpoints about us being lazy or crazy.

At my next immunology appointment, Dr Spickett was away. Instead, I saw a specialist registrar. He wanted to put me back on Aciclovir even though I wasn't currently going through a full relapse. I explained I usually only went on the drugs when I was IgM positive, but the registrar wanted to find out what was happening to my body between relapses. He told me to stay on a low dose of Aciclovir while he did a PCR test to see if I still had EBV DNA in my blood. PCR testing was not commonplace at the time (of course, Covid has changed all that), and I was excited to be undergoing a process I had learnt about at university.

As he chatted enthusiastically about the test, I momentarily felt like I was back at a lecture. But it turns out that being under a microscope isn't half as much fun as looking down one. At times like that, I felt on the wrong side of life.

When the results came back a few weeks later, they showed I did still have EBV DNA in my blood (and also atypical monocytes). In other words, the glandular fever was active in my system in between – as well as during – my relapses. I'm trying not to overdramatise here, but those results honestly changed my life. The remaining doubters had to accept now that I had a continual, long-term viral infection, and not just an empty petrol tank.

The registrar asked me to stay on low-dose Aciclovir for several months, and I slowly improved to the point of being able to do half an hour of activity each day.

Meaning I could get back to my nutrition course. Hurrah!

Because of my ill health, it had taken me four and a half years to get two-thirds of the way through my diploma. As I mentioned previously, students were given five years to finish the course, but the organisers had agreed to extend this in my case. Unfortunately, at that time there was a change in leadership. The college principal had died, and his wife was in pieces, so a new set of staff swooped in to take over. They didn't know me from Eve. And, of course, I had no written evidence that the old principal had said I could do the diploma at my own rate.

I was told that I had to complete the course promptly. I argued my case, but I'm not sure the new staff believed me. The only concession they made was to offer me an additional six months 'as a gesture of goodwill'. I hit the books hard, pushing myself through the brain fog to answer question after question. But my glandular fever was quick to protest. I had to be realistic. It had taken me four and a half years to finish twenty-four modules; I could no more do twelve modules in twelve months than I could run twelve marathons in twelve days.

With no other choice, I was forced to call the college and drop out. Everything that I had worked for had come to nothing. There was no silver medal for completing *most* of the course.

I was inconsolable. In my quest for a career, I had tried everything to accommodate my illness, from changing universities to reducing my hours. But the glandular fever refused to compromise. The nutrition diploma had been my hope, my way out, my chance at a normal life. I had had it all planned out; I was going to run my practice from my conservatory. I knew where I would put my desk, where the patient would sit, everything. It had been my future.

Except now it wasn't.

Chapter 15

I once read that we are each genetically programmed to experience a certain range of happiness and sadness. It was at this point in my life that I discovered the lowest point of my own scale. But being at rock bottom brings out my determined side, and I resolved to turn things around. There was no way I was going to live the rest of my life as a half-wraith.

First, though, I needed a realistic prognosis for my illness. I'd asked for one previously from my immunologists, of course, but they'd always given me evasive answers – except for once when I'd been told I had less chance of getting fully better than I did of winning the lottery. I'd tried to do my own research, but I couldn't find any useful prognoses for sufferers of ME/CFS with ongoing viral symptoms such as mine. For example, in one of my guides from that time, *Living With ME*, the section on recovery rates stated that ME/CFS sufferers with repeated infections (like me) 'probably don't do so well'. Talk about demoralising.

But now, nearing the end of my twenties and with yet another career plan quashed by my illness, I needed to know where I was headed. My PCR result had led to a subtle shift in diagnosis away from ME/CFS to a state of 'chronic EBV'.

So perhaps I should try Googling the outcomes of sufferers with that label? Maybe then I'd find a happy ending?

Feeling optimistic, I opened my web browser, typed in 'chronic EBV', and clicked on one of the links.

The article[a] started: *Chronic Active Epstein-Barr Virus infection (CAEBV) is a high-mortality and high-morbidity disease—*

Panicked, I flicked the computer screen off.

That statement put a whole new complexion on my situation. 'High mortality' isn't a term you ever want to read concerning yourself. Previously, I had assumed the worst thing about my illness was not knowing when or how I would recover. Now, I realised I might not recover at all.

Plucking up courage, I turned the screen back on. The rest of the article (a Japanese study) wasn't as terrifying as the first sentence had been. It went on to explain that CAEBV in the Western hemisphere is usually milder than in Japan. And from this and the next few papers I read, I learnt that chronic glandular fever is not so much one illness as a range of conditions extending from 'Severe Chronic Active EBV' at one extreme (the type that's often lethal) to 'Chronic EBV' at the other (the type that's less serious).

Unfortunately, working out precisely where I fell on this scale was an impossible task. For starters, many articles adopted muddled terminology, using 'Chronic Active EBV' to mean everything from the most to the least severe kind of the illness. More importantly, my personal physiological responses to EBV (for example, my antibody levels and organ involvement) varied in their severity, putting some of my results on the positive end of the scale, and others on the negative.

If there was one thing clear, though, it was that my symptoms weren't anywhere near as serious as those poor souls with the severest form of the illness. That discovery was a pivotal moment in my life because it made me feel that I was one of the lucky ones.

Relieved, I resolved to make the most of what health I had rather than always wanting more. Odds were, I would never manage to fight off the virus completely, so I would most likely spend the rest of my life alternating between a little bit ill and very ill. As a result, I had to accept I probably wouldn't have a career. I told myself that I was fine about this, and that instead of finding a job I would have to spend my life doing… doing…

Doing what?

I felt like I was having a midlife crisis twenty years early. If I wasn't a scientist or a nutritionist, who was I?

Strange how often we define ourselves by what we do instead of who we are.

*

A few nights later, I was lying awake in bed, turning over these thoughts in my head, when I realised I couldn't keep them to myself any more. I prodded Jon softly.

'I need to talk to you.'

He groaned, but his eyes remained shut. 'What time is it?'

'Just after four.'

'What's happened?'

'I can't sleep. I need to ask you something.'

Finally, he opened his eyes, and I felt guilty when I saw the black shadows beneath them. 'If you had to describe me in three words – and this is important – what would those three words be?'

I could tell he didn't know whether to be amused or annoyed. 'I have to answer this at four in the morning?'

'Yes.'

'Why?'

'Because I won't be able to sleep until you do.'

He studied my face closely. I must have looked pretty harrowed because he agreed to this crazy request. After some thought, he mumbled, 'I'm afraid I'm too tired to think of three things. But the first word to describe you, your best quality, that's easy. If I tell you that, can we go back to sleep?'

'OK.'

'Courageous.'

'What? How can you think I'm courageous? I'm scared of everything!'

'Like what?'

'Like every time I step on a plane, I'm convinced I'm going to die.'

'But you fly anyway.'

'And that time I had to go into the CT scanner at the RVI – you know, when I was having all those tests – I felt so claustrophobic, I almost freaked out.'

'But you didn't. You let them do the scan.'

I stared at Jon, unable to get my head around what he was saying. I had never considered myself brave, yet here was Jon saying it was my main trait. I wanted to discuss it further, but Jon reminded me of our agreement. 'I've given you my answer,' he said. 'It's sleep time.'

I wrapped myself around him, and he closed his eyes.

When his breathing slowed, I rolled over to my side

of the bed and got up. I walked over to the window and stayed there until the sun started to rise. I watched the birds flittering in and out of the hedges; the milkman delivering bottles to the house on the corner; then, later, front doors opening as neighbours left for work. You can't stop the world from turning. If Jon was right, if I truly were courageous, then I would have to quit worrying about who I was now and let tomorrow take care of itself.

The following afternoon we were sharing the big sofa in the lounge. Jon was reading the paper, and I was horizontal as usual, my head resting on his lap. Suddenly, Jon put the paper down and said, 'OK, I've managed to whittle it down to four, but I can't get it any lower.'

'What are you talking about?'

'The words that describe you.'

'You've actually been thinking about it?' Jon usually forgets everything we discuss in the early hours. Or any hours, for that matter.

'Of course,' he said. 'But first I'm curious to know how you see yourself.'

'I have no idea any more,' I replied, pushing myself upright. 'That's the problem. So, what did you come up with?'

He gave a half-smile. 'Is this the part where I tell you how attractive and intelligent you are?'

'A girl can dream.'

He grabbed my hand. 'Lily, there are thousands of attractive and intelligent women out there.' He pointed out the window as if they were all lined up on our street. 'I thought you wanted to know what made you unique.'

I wasn't sure I liked him thinking there were *thousands* of attractive women around, but decided this wasn't the time to discuss it. 'All I mean is, everyone has their "thing", don't they? Mine has always been science.' I looked away. 'I can just about handle the illness taking my social life and my physical health. But I can't come to terms with it taking the science. Because that's what makes me *me*.'

'No, it isn't,' said Jon. And he went on to explain the other qualities that had made his top four – lovely characteristics that I admire in others and aspire to have myself. I wondered if I should remove Jon's rose-tinted spectacles or, for the sake of our marriage, just let him keep them on.

'So… is that why you fell in love with me?' I asked.

He went back to his newspaper. 'No,' he said, his wry smile returning. 'I fell for your IQ score.'

*

'Can I come in or are you resting?' It was my mum, calling around with two carrier bags full of clean laundry.

I told her she could come through. 'I was awake half the night, so I should be in bed,' I said. 'But it's lovely to see you.'

'Half the night?' she enquired as she took off her jacket.

I hesitated, unsure whether to tell her. 'Yes,' I said eventually. 'I had this crazy notion of waking Jon at four in the morning to ask him what words define me.'

'Ooh! Let me think!'

'No, really,' I said, already regretting mentioning it. 'It was silly of me.'

But my protests were ignored.

Mum frowned as she deliberated. 'You're… you're…'

I wondered what was coming. What do mothers usually

say about their daughters? That they're thoughtful? Caring? Affectionate?

'I know!' she declared. 'You're a hoot!'

'What?'

Mum's face fell. 'You're offended.'

'I'm... surprised.'

'I meant it as a compliment. Why, what did Jon come up with?'

'He said I was courageous.'

'Oh! That's even more true. Yes, I take mine back. I'm saying courageous too.'

'You can't do that!' I objected. 'You can't withdraw your answer and steal someone else's.'

'But it's better.'

'That's not the point!'

It was time to change the topic, so I moved the conversation on to more intellectual things like the Eurovision Song Contest and whether anything in the world was cuter than a baby guinea pig. But you can only hide your demons from your mother for so long. Soon I was explaining to her that I only felt like 'me' when I was studying or researching, and she huffed about how unfairly the nutrition college had treated me.

The next day I was having breakfast with Jon when there was a tentative knock at the front door. It was Mum again.

'I didn't want to disturb you two days in a row,' she said. 'But I was thinking last night about what I said. Can I come in?' Inside, she cleared her throat. 'When I called you a hoot, and you were offended...'

'Mum, how many times? I was just surprised.'

'You were offended. I can tell these things.'

'Because you're a psychiatrist?'

'Because I'm your mother. Anyway, I wanted to explain. I didn't mean that you were a laughingstock. People actually admire you, you know.'

'*Now* you're sounding like my mother.'

'Shush, I'm trying to explain. What I mean is, you have a quality of making others happy.'

For a moment, I couldn't speak. How could anyone say that about me? There I was, in my skanky dressing gown, moping about my career plans going down the drain. Only yesterday I'd needed Jon's reassurances to cheer me up. If I couldn't even make *myself* happy, how happy could I possibly make others?

Seeing I was unconvinced, Mum added, 'It's true. We could ask anyone who has ever met you, "How did you feel after you spoke to Lily?" and they would say, "Happier".'

'Oh, Mum, you're so sweet.'

'You don't believe me? I'll call everyone up now. Whom shall I ring first?' She got up and strode towards the phone. Her face had a determined cast to it, but she had to be calling my bluff. I was… almost certain of it.

I darted for the phone and grabbed it before she did. 'I believe you think that,' I said. 'But I don't know how you can, when I've been such a misery.'

'Well, it's true,' she said.

As she departed, Jon came in to ask what that had all been about. When I explained about the 'hoot' comment, he said, 'She probably just meant you're a character. That runs in the family.'

Neither Jon nor Mum remembers those conversations. Nor did they appreciate the effect their words had on me. The stories of Mum crying at church, and in the lay-by outside the pub, had made me feel like a killjoy, yet here she was telling me that I made her happier. I wish I had realised that sooner.

More importantly, the qualities in me that Jon had fallen in love with were traits that had either been created, or intensified, by my illness. If I really possessed those characteristics, then the illness had not been all bad. It had made me a better person.

*

I had been ignoring my biological clock for a while now, so I decided it was time to address it. At my next appointment with Dr Spickett, I asked him what effect the immune shifts associated with pregnancy could have on my fragile health. He told me there was no way of knowing; I could end up worse, better, or I could stay the same.

Nice to have that cleared up.

I asked if I would be able to go on Aciclovir while I was pregnant, and he said no. At that time, it was believed it might affect the foetus. I quizzed him on whether he thought it was right for me to bring a child into the world. By that I meant, was it fair for the child to have a mother with my physical limitations? He told me I should stop thinking so much and go with my heart.

But my heart didn't know what it wanted, so for several weeks I let my head take the wheel. I imagined myself on my death bed. Cheery thinking, I know, but it was effective for establishing my priorities. I decided that, by the time I reached the end of my life, I wanted, above all else, to have done two things. The first was to write a book so I could make the world understand ME/CFS properly. The second was to try for a baby.

I went to my GP and asked for a referral to an obstetrician. After years of illness, I needed to know how my polycystic ovaries were doing. The obstetrician said that my immune system, rather than my ovaries, would be the deciding factor in whether I had a successful pregnancy. She also pointed out that if I managed to have a baby, the child – like all kids – would pick up a constant stream of infections for the first five years or so. And, of course, I would catch them from him or her. How would my immune system cope with that?

She had a point, but by this time my mind was made up. I had to try. I said to Jon, 'If my health stays the same or gets worse, and I'm never well enough to run with our child or roll down hills with it in the summer, will you do all that? Will you be the mad, silly one?'

'I always assumed you'd be the crazy parent and I'd bring a bit of sense to the family,' he replied.

'You know what I'm getting at. Will you play with it and fling it about? A kid needs that.'

He pretended to consider. 'Act like a child myself, you mean? Hmm… If you insist.'

'Then I think we'll go for it. Not yet, though. First I have to sort out my internal biochemistry.'

He gave me an odd look. 'You do that,' he said.

*

Before I tried to conceive, I needed to see if I could wean myself off my antihistamines and elderberry extract. I really wanted to have a medicine-free pregnancy (apart from my thyroid pills, which I was on for life). To replace the antihistamines, I took fish oil daily.[4] After several months, it calmed down my allergic responses enough for me to come off the antihistamines completely. My joint pains also improved.

Unfortunately, cutting out the elderberry extract was a different matter. All the articles I read said that elderberry might not be safe in pregnancy. However, when I tried coming off the pills, my viral symptoms worsened. What was I supposed to do? Taking elderberry posed a risk to the baby, but *not* taking it might prove equally dangerous. Because whilst Dr Spickett assured me low levels of EBV posed no danger to a foetus, no one knew what the effects of a full-blown relapse would be.

While I tried to unpick this knot, I turned my attention to writing this book. I had always vented about my illness in my diary – so much so, I almost felt sorry for it – so I had a good record of the main events. Then I started keeping a pack of Post-it notes beside my bed, and whenever I heard someone say something untrue or uninformed about my illness, I scribbled it down. Meanwhile, events from my past were returning to me on a daily basis. I jotted these things down too and soon found I had at least one scene that demonstrated each point I wanted to make.

The next day, I spread out all of the Post-it notes on

---

4 A person's immune state can be influenced by the balance of omega-3 and omega-6 fatty acids in their diet. I had already improved my health by reducing foods high in the latter (mostly greasy, beige foods) and taking fish oil when I could face it. Now, for a few months, I tried to eat little or no 'bad fats', as well as taking the maximum dose of the purest fish oil daily. (By 'purest' I mean one that is free from pollutants such as PCBs, and that comes from oily fish at the bottom of the food chain rather than large predatory fish which are more likely to contain higher levels of heavy metals. I also mean fish oil and not cod liver oil, which is very high in vitamin A and therefore best avoided by women in pregnancy.)

the carpet in the spare bedroom and organised them into chapters. I had never before written anything as long as a book, but I was determined to do it even if it took me twenty years. I wanted other sufferers to learn not just from what had worked for me, but also from my mistakes. And the doctors who treated the condition too, surely they would be interested in my story? Because even the ones who acknowledge ME/CFS as a real illness don't always feel confident about treating it. (I know this from reading Mum's beloved medical magazines.)

For the next few weeks, I wrote every day that I could. I would manage only fifteen minutes before my brain fog descended, but, word by word, I inched towards my target. Once I had finished chapter one in its first draft, I knew that this was my vocation. Nothing, absolutely nothing, was going to stop me from finishing it.

Then I rushed to the bathroom and vomited.

Chapter 16

Yes, that's right, I was pregnant. When the tests confirmed it, I floated around the house with one hand constantly stroking my belly. Even Jon displayed a touch of exuberance. I stopped taking elderberry and waited anxiously for the glandular fever to flare up. But, instead, I felt less viral than I had for the past twelve years. The immune shifts caused by my pregnancy appeared to have dampened down the EBV. My brain fog was all but gone. For the first time in my adult life, I felt 'back in the room'. I didn't need elderberry any more!

But the bugs were already planning their next attack. It was November, so I couldn't step outside my house without a stranger coughing on me. And now that I was pregnant, I was more susceptible to infections than ever. In those early weeks, most of my time was spent shivering in bed, or waiting in the surgery for a doctor to listen to the crackles in my chest. Things weren't exactly going to plan. When my friends had fallen pregnant, their talk had been all about the baby's gender and future name. My conversations were about mucus and body temperature.

One thing the doctors impressed upon me was that I

had to look after myself. The trouble was, Christmas was looming, and I was due to go down to Nottingham to spend it with Jon's family. Then we found out that one of his nephews had flu, and that his sister had just been discharged from hospital after suffering from norovirus. If I mixed with them, I was sure to catch what they had, and if that precipitated a glandular fever relapse, the baby might be harmed. I told Jon to go without me, but he refused to leave me alone over the festive season. So, he phoned his parents to explain we might not be there.

His mum and dad urged us to come. They said Jon's sister shouldn't be contagious by the time we arrived, and that I could stay away from the ill nephew. My mother-in-law even suggested we all wear face masks to inhibit the spread of the viruses. This was long before the pandemic, so I was impressed by her initiative. But I wasn't convinced that surgical masks would help everyone get into the Christmas spirit.

Nonetheless, I was touched by the lengths they were prepared to go to to accommodate me, and I decided that I couldn't *not* go.

So, on Christmas Eve, we arrived at my in-laws' house. My nephew tottered to the door to greet me with two green tracks streaming from his nostrils. My poor sister-in-law was too ill to get up; I found her lying on the lounge sofa with a bucket beside her. I could almost sense the bugs lining up to take a shot at me, but I resigned myself to the inevitable and tried to relax. Then my mother-in-law suggested moving in with me and Jon when the baby was born.

I had to decline. Many other women would have welcomed the offer of assistance with their newborn, but for someone with my illness, having a guest – even a family member – just makes you sicker. You can't rest properly, your sleep is interrupted, and you feel you should chat when you're only well enough to grunt. I wouldn't be able to cope with anyone staying at what would already be the most physically demanding time of my life.

It must have seemed like I was being unaccommodating. I felt frustrated at myself for being unable to explain my limitations properly. At times like that, my urge to write would become overwhelming.

'I wish I were working on my book,' I confessed to Jon when we were alone later.

He smiled. 'But back at home, you said you weren't going to write your book now you're pregnant,' he teased me. 'I distinctly remember the conversation.'

I remembered it too. I had told Jon I wouldn't have the health to write *and* look after a child.

'Lily,' he went on. 'You've been happier writing your first chapter than I've seen you in years. You have to keep going.'

That night, I lay awake for hours. My mind kept turning over. I had too many concerns to juggle: my pregnancy, my book, the expectations of family – not to mention the EBV. I tried to think of a way to make this work for everyone without damaging my health.

Eventually, I forced myself to focus on the baby. Some women need to see their child before they feel a connection to it, but I loved my foetus from the moment it was conceived. I used to chat to it each day, much to Jon's amusement. It was that love that finally lulled me to sleep.

*

When I awoke on Christmas morning, my throat felt like I had swallowed a sprig of holly. But seeing Jon so bright eyed helped to lift my mood.

'Can't wait for you to open your presents,' he said. He seemed suspiciously eager at the prospect.

'You've not got me something good, have you, babe?'

Most wives would have been thrilled at the thought of an exciting present coming their way. But I felt the opposite because I hadn't had the health to find a special gift for Jon. Somewhere between my first midwife appointment and my third respiratory tract infection I had ordered him some swanky pyjamas from the internet. But now I feared that the only positive thing you could say about them was that they weren't socks.

'I haven't bought you anything expensive, if that's what you mean,' Jon replied. Then, 'I think we had better make ourselves decent. Sounds like things have started down there.'

He was right. Judging by the giggles, shrieks and electronic toy music coming from downstairs, the others had been up for a while. So, we showered, applied antiviral cream to our hands (in an attempt to fend off norovirus), and headed down to join the masses.

Towards the end of the present opening, I found a mysterious parcel from Jon. He and his smile joined me on the sofa while I tore off the paper. It felt like a book, but why would he be so pleased with himself over that? Then I saw the title: *Your Life As Story*. It said on the front cover that it was a 'sourcebook for all writers interested in putting their life stories down on paper'. In other words, a guide to help me write this book. I grinned at him, and for a second it seemed like we were the only two people in the room.

'Are you trying to tell me something?' I asked.

'I spent weeks searching for the right book,' he replied. 'I couldn't find any that dealt specifically with writing about illness, but the reviews for that one were good.'

'I love it!' I said, welling up. 'I think you're the only person who hasn't given up on me.'

'Maybe that's because I'm the one who knows you best.'

Then Jon crawled under the Christmas tree and grabbed a gold-wrapped gift before passing it to me. 'Here you go.'

I peeled off the sticky tape at the top. I was expecting to find a piece of jewellery inside until I saw from the box that it was something electronic. Strange. Jon knew I didn't like gadgets. Feeling sceptical, I removed the rest of the paper to find…

'A Dictaphone!'

'It's for the days when you are too ill to write,' Jon explained. 'You can dictate your book ideas onto that, then type them up when you're feeling better.'

There can't be many wives who cry when the small, cuboid present from their husband turns out to be a Dictaphone – not tears of happiness, at least. But I loved what it signified: that Jon thought I could get my book written; that he understood what I needed to do with my life; and that he wasn't prepared to let me give up on my ambition.

I wanted the same for Jon, too. Recently, we had started talking about his own goals, and he told me what I had already known: he wasn't happy in his career. Back in my Cambridge days, he'd told me animatedly that he wrote fiction in his free time, and I knew then that he was in the wrong job. I guess I had been waiting eleven years for him to work it out for himself.

Now, he wanted more time to write, and since I would need help looking after our baby, the solution seemed obvious: Jon would reduce the hours he worked at his firm and split his newly acquired free time between writing and helping me at home.

Our minds made up, we told our respective families about our plans. Naively, we had expected them to share our enthusiasm. But their stiff smiles failed to conceal their reservations. Whilst Jon and I understood our families' concerns, we knew that something in our lives had to change. Every morning, Jon left me alone in bed with a fever to go to a job he didn't enjoy, to earn money for a life that I was too ill to experience with him. That did not work for either of us, nor was it the right set-up for bringing a child into the world.

*

We arrived home from our Christmas trip with an extra present: our nephew's bug. January saw us both in bed with high temperatures just as my morning sickness was taking hold. The two conditions joined forces to tag team me. When I lay down, I couldn't breathe through my nose, but when I propped myself up on my pillows, the sickness came surging back. And yet, I still felt so much better than I had for the past twelve years. One morning, I sat up to explain this to Jon, who was lying beside me. But instead, I found myself projectile vomiting onto his pyjama top – the one I'd bought him for Christmas.

As January came to a close, it was time for my twelve-week scan. There was a delay at the hospital. I was sitting with Jon in the packed waiting room for ages, listening to the babies babbling and crying all around us. A girl was opposite us, sucking her thumb as her mother read to her, while behind her a boy smeared in chocolate zoomed around like a Duracell bunny with an extra battery. I wondered which of the two my own child would resemble. A quiet one would be easier on me physically, but in truth I didn't mind. Somehow, I would find a way to cope.

Eventually, it was my turn to be scanned. I lay on the couch with the cold gel on my tummy, Jon holding my hand as the sonographer moved her scanner over my abdomen. I saw the baby's snubbed nose and tiny fingers, and I felt such a rush of maternal love. I wanted to reach out and touch the screen. I had seen baby scan photos before, of course, and I had wondered at the gushy reactions they elicited in others. But seeing your own child for the first time is… staggering. The baby meant everything to me.

Then I saw the sonographer's face, and I realised something was wrong. Studying the screen more closely, I quickly spotted the problem. I grasped Jon's hand more tightly. He was still smiling, totally unaware of what was going on. I looked frantically from him to the sonographer and back again, wanting him to hear it from me, but finding myself unable to speak.

Then the sonographer said calmly, sorrowfully, 'I'm so sorry. I can't find a heartbeat.'

*

The baby had died recently, but my body still thought I was pregnant. I chose what is termed 'medical management' to expel the foetus and was told to come back to hospital the next day. As the nurses gave me the Prostaglandin drug, I felt lost, vulnerable, scared. And when the first contractions came, all I could think was, *this is not how my first labour should be.* I was told not to look as the foetus was being delivered, and I really tried not to. But I did catch a glimpse of the small, perfectly formed body, the tiny bones visible through translucent skin. It struck me then that the difference between life and death is just the flick of a biological switch.

For several days afterwards, I lay in the spare room at home with a towel underneath me, staring at nothing. My immune system had reset to its pre-pregnancy state, and the glandular fever had flared up again. Jon would come home from his half-day at the office and lie beside me. He played 'Chasing Cars' by Snow Patrol on the CD player, and we would lie with our arms round each other and listen to Gary Lightbody sing about forgetting the world. But I couldn't forget the world, however much I wanted to.

Then one day, I noticed a rainbow outside, and something clicked within me. I know it sounds cheesy, but I realised the phases of my life were like the bands of that rainbow – some bright, others dark, yet each one adding to the whole. Take any one of them away and I wouldn't be the same person I was. Remove the blue, and the red wouldn't look so vibrant.

Jon and I decided to escape to the Champagne region of France. We drowned our sorrows in bubbly, took long drives through the vineyards, and reassured ourselves that the baby-and-book dream was still possible. Then we lit a candle for our lost child in Reims Cathedral and returned to Durham, ready to move on.

When word got around about my miscarriage, a steady flow of people came to see me. I was truly grateful for their kind words and flowers, yet a part of me wondered where their empathy had been throughout the twelve years of my illness. Could they not relate to my disability in the way they could my miscarriage?

I don't want to downplay the loss of my baby. Chronic illness is not worse than a miscarriage, just different. It isn't a single event. The ME/CFS was my daily grind, unceasing and relentless. You can move on from many of life's tragedies, but you cannot fully move on from something that has no end.

*

After my miscarriage, I felt older, more resilient and able to tackle anything. That included trying for another child. So, three months later I found myself with my head down the toilet again, vomiting up what little food I had managed to force down. Unfortunately, where the previous pregnancy had temporarily suppressed my glandular fever, this one made it worse. By taking care of myself, I kept the virus at a low level without needing to resort to medication. Yet I still looked forward eagerly to the day that I went into labour – and there can't be many women who say that.

I spent nearly every second of every day flat out with a virus or sprinting to the bathroom to be sick – but at least that meant I was getting some exercise. On the day of the dating scan, my nerves gave me another reason to feel queasy. When the image of my child came up on the screen, the first thing the doctor said was, 'Look at its long legs!' But all I could focus on was its heart, beating away. 'You've got a lively one,' she said.

I could breathe again.

As far as things like blood pressure, bump growth and iron levels were concerned, I was having a healthy pregnancy. At my check-ups, the midwife always told me she was glad to see me, because I guaranteed her a short appointment and thus time to catch up with her schedule. This was quite a turnaround for the girl whose medical complications had always caused her doctors to run late.

Back at home, I was too ill to read, so Jon flicked through an entire maternity book and flagged the important bits for me. One day, at the seven-month stage, I opened my eyes to find him hovering over the bed. He told me what he'd learnt about ideal nursery temperatures and the tog ratings of sleeping bags. At the sound of his voice, the baby kicked. When Jon gently tapped it through my skin, the baby responded by punching the spot that Jon was tapping.

'Look,' he said. 'We're communicating!'

'It's hardly Morse code, babe,' I replied. But secretly I was delighted at their interaction.

Most of the women in my life wanted a piece of me while I was pregnant. They kept ringing to ask me what pram we were getting or why we weren't having a baby shower. They complained that we weren't involving them in the pregnancy, but if shopping for prams and cots was their definition of that, I wasn't involved in my pregnancy either. Almost eight months in, Jon said we had to get on with the essentials. It was time to turn our home office into a nursery.

The room had a huge built-in cupboard containing the remains of my healthy life: files and science textbooks, practical notes from my experiments at Cambridge... remnants of an overzealous, idealistic student. I had novels, too – classics, my beloved Aldous Huxleys – all of which I was now too ill to read. I reached to the back of the cupboard and pulled out my old Cambridge gown, slightly musty, underused. Next came my nutrition course files, my school certificates, tiny trophies from my dancing days. There was even a photo of me on skis in the Alps, grinning in my pink headband and sunglasses.

It was crushing, demoralising, sifting through those lost dreams. I wanted to clear it all immediately, but I was so ill I could only rehouse two items at a time. Later, on the good days, it became three. Towards the end of the process, I realised that I had not just sorted through the cupboard, I had sorted through my old life as well. Cleared away the mental baggage I had been carrying for the past thirteen years. Forget about the pram-buying and the baby shower, *this* was the most important thing I could have done in readiness for my child's birth. I needed to create a fresh start for myself so I did not go into motherhood scarred by my past. I was ready now for him to be born.

Yes, I did say 'him', because by this stage I knew it was a boy. As my due date approached, I realised I had missed all except one of my antenatal classes due to illness, but I finally felt well enough for a visitor. Caja was quick to come around. Bless her, she had not hassled me at all for the past nine months because she knew how hard it was to be pregnant with ME/CFS – she was pregnant herself at that time. She brought me baby gifts: bright board books with different textures and just a couple of huge words on each page. Even with my brain fog, I figured I would manage to read my child these.

*

Twelve days past my due date. Twelve days of calls and texts from relatives and friends demanding, 'Have you had the baby yet?'

That night, I was heaving myself into bed when: 'Argghh!'

'You OK up there?' Jon called from the lounge below.

'No, I think…'

But you really can't talk when there's a baby trying to exit. Or at least not in a language that anyone who hasn't experienced labour can understand.

Jon phoned the hospital, loaded the car, came back into the house and—

'What on earth are you doing?' he asked me.

I was holding a J-cloth and Ecover spray. 'Getting the place decent for your parents,' I explained. I had agreed to let them stay for one night after the baby was born. And I don't know if it was because of my hormones, or because my illness had trained me to push through physical discomfort, but I managed to ignore those first contractions long enough to get the bathroom gleaming.

*

I staggered down the hospital corridor, leaning against the wall with every contraction. When I finally made it to the examination room, the midwife inspected me to see how dilated I was.

'Three centimetres,' she declared.

'What?' From the books I'd read, I knew that three centimetres meant I was probably about seven hours away from showtime. But that's not what my body was telling me. 'I must be further on than that,' I added. 'These contractions are coming every min—' I broke off as the next one rose inside me. Throughout it, I chanted something internally that I had learnt from my convalescence: *this too shall pass, this too shall pass…*

'What's she doing?' the midwife asked Jon.

'Er, having a contraction?' he replied, clearly surprised – and a little concerned – that she needed to be told.

'I'll get her some paracetamol,' the woman said dismissively as she rinsed her hands at the sink. 'Then you can go home. Maybe come back tomorrow.'

'Paracetamol helps *these*?' I asked in disbelief, wondering why my birthing manual hadn't mentioned that.

'Of course,' the midwife said, disappearing through the door.

'I'm much further along than she thinks,' I told Jon. 'I can feel him coming. The pain is unbeliev—' But I couldn't finish the sentence.

'Then we're not going anywhere,' replied Jon.

The midwife returned to drop off the pills and said I could stay until they started working. But they could have been Tic Tacs for all the effect they had. I was in so much pain I thought my body would explode.

Then it got worse. During my contractions, I closed my eyes and visualised myself leaping over hurdles. I didn't even notice when the midwife returned later.

'Is the paracetamol working?' she asked.

I waited until the break between contractions to say, 'There must be some mistake. I can feel the baby coming.'

She appeared not to hear me. 'Maybe a hot bath at home might help.'

Go home? I wasn't even able to walk. The baby was on

his way, but only Jon seemed to believe me. As I escaped back into my head to jump hurdles, I felt a crushing pain. My waters had broken.

The midwife rushed over, her expression turning swiftly from panic to efficiency. She shouted something out of the door, then strapped a monitor onto me to check the baby's heartbeat. The colour of the fluid had indicated it contained meconium, signalling the baby was in distress. Visions of a second dead child darted through my mind.

'I'll just see how things are going,' said the midwife. Then a startled, 'Oh my, he's right here!' As if I hadn't spent the last hour trying to tell her that. 'Does your husband want to see his scalp?'

'Not especially,' muttered Jon, staying resolutely at my head end.

Finally, the midwife offered me some gas and air. Then a more senior midwife entered the room, together with a young male paediatrician who paced up and down, not knowing where to look. Despite the contractions, I was alert enough to realise this was not routine.

'Is there something wrong with my baby?' I panted.

But I didn't hear the answer because the next thing I knew, I was wailing like a banshee as my son was delivered. A couple of cries showed his displeasure at being brought into this bright, noisy world. Then his cord was cut, and our son Matty was passed to me in a swaddled bundle.

His huge blue eyes searched through their haze to find mine. The instant our gazes met, he seemed to settle, as if he recognised me. I held him tightly and drank in his features. One of the midwives joked, 'Well, there's no doubt who the father is!' And she was right: Matty resembled a mini-Jon. I found myself grinning with relief because he looked so well. In the back of my mind, I'd always been aware that my illness could have affected his development in the womb. EBV had blighted my life; I didn't want it scarring his as well.

The paediatrician checked Matty over and confirmed he was indeed healthy. Then Jon got his first chance to hold him, and the two of them spent minutes staring at each other, spellbound. After the senior midwife left with the paediatrician, I was told I would need minor surgery and so I lay back to wait for the obstetrician.

Shortly afterwards, my mum appeared, expecting to find me still in labour. When she saw Matty in Jon's arms, she did a double take then rushed over to check on us. The midwife, meanwhile, was shuffling around my bed, clearing up. She couldn't look me in the eye. When she finally finished, she took a couple of steps towards the door before stopping and swinging around. She took a deep breath, then said, 'You're the bravest woman I have ever delivered a baby for.'

I forced a smile. 'Bet you say that to everyone.'

'No, I don't.'

Her eyes were full of guilt for not believing me when I told her Matty was on his way. I felt sorry for her. 'You were great,' I lied.

But that only seemed to make her feel worse.

The moment was broken by the arrival of the obstetrician. She flinched when she heard that I hadn't had an epidural.

'But I did have some paracetamol,' I said.

My comment made the midwife blush, so I hurriedly mentioned the gas and air she had provided me with at the end.

While the obstetrician got to work, I thought of what the

midwife had said to me. I wasn't brave. Every week, there are hundreds of women who endure far more traumatic births than mine. And anyway, for someone with a long-term illness, times like that are just another day at the office. By that I mean you live with discomfort on a daily basis, and you try to explain how you feel to medical professionals, who, if you're lucky, might listen to what you're telling them. But all too often they simply stick to what they believe instead, like the midwife had. What can you do, though? You just have to get on with it.

I wonder if the way the midwife felt at the end – the guilt, the realisation that I had been going through something worse than she had thought – will be how people feel when they start to understand this illness. But I don't want them to feel guilty. I just want them to hear.

Chapter 17

Matty was a happy child, but he was *so* lively. 'Does he ever stop?' a midwife once asked me, and I honestly couldn't think of a time when he wasn't bouncing or kicking or flapping his arms about. All this activity meant he needed extra food – more than I could provide him with through breastfeeding alone. So, Jon had to top him up with formula milk, meaning we were both involved in every feed, day and night. Then Matty would vomit it all up again just in time for the next meal to begin.

Soon his health started to deteriorate. He developed eczema and an abdomen so bloated he looked like the kids on the news with kwashiorkor. Eventually, a paediatric immunologist diagnosed oesophageal reflux and a cow's milk allergy.

Unfortunately, that marked just the beginning of Matty's health problems. So often did we have to take him to our local hospital with a sky-high fever, we were ultimately given open access to the children's ward. One after another, Matty developed cystitis, tonsillitis, bronchiolitis… At times, it felt like he was working his way through every '*itis*' in the medical dictionary.

Friends and relatives started complaining that they weren't getting enough fun time with Matty. They didn't realise we weren't getting much either. People used to ask me which mother-and-baby group I was going to, or which baby swim classes I was considering. I wouldn't know how to answer, because even when Matty was well, *I* wasn't. Not once did I have the health to push Matty in his buggy. I fed him, I sang to him, I read to him until my inflamed pharynx could take no more. But I was never a normal mum.

Matty would snuggle into my dressing gown as I worked my way through a pile of children's library books. I remember his concentrated expression as he tried to follow the words on the page. Board books with a few words turned into paper books as Matty made the transition from babyhood to toddlerhood. Once, while I was reading him a rhyming book called *Let's Take Over The Nursery!* Matty got the giggles, which then set me off too. The memory of the two of us doubled up laughing has carried me through many hard times.

*

Throughout this period, my health was sliding relentlessly downhill. Eventually my check-up with Dr Spickett came around, and a blood test confirmed I was back in the acute stages of glandular fever. It was a relief to go on the high-dose Aciclovir. I felt that I could finally start recovering.

Then one evening I found a hard, immobile lump in my breast.

I had thought that being ill for a decade and a half would have prepared me for every eventuality, but the head-spin you get when you think you might have cancer is something else entirely. No matter how rational you force yourself to be, your brain keeps seeing flashes of a tombstone with your name on it.

I looked up the lump on the internet, but it didn't seem to fit the description of anything that wasn't serious. I discussed it over and over with Jon, hoping that the more I spoke about it, the more my mind would find an innocent explanation. I mean, there was no history of breast cancer in my family. None. How many women can say that? But then it occurred to me that having a viral infection for fifteen years would increase the odds of the Big C. I googled to see if breast cancer was one of the diseases EBV was associated with.

It was.

I lay awake all night worrying.

The following morning, Jon drove me to the doctor's surgery. I was too nervous to speak and spent the journey in stony silence while Matty was in the back, humming the tune to 'The Sun Has Got His Hat On'.

At the surgery, it seemed like the world was moving in slow motion as patients trooped in and out with their coughs and limps. When I was eventually called in, I gabbled to the doctor and prayed for the all-clear. Initially she chirped some reassurances based on my age and family history. But when she felt the lump, her tone faltered. And as she checked the glands under my armpit, there was only one explanation for her sudden faux breeziness: she definitely thought it was cancer. I asked her outright, 'Do you?'

She said, 'It certainly ticks all the boxes for a very urgent referral.'

Two days later, I was assessed by a specialist. Then

two days after *that*, I went for a scan at the breast clinic at Queen Elizabeth Hospital in Gateshead. As I filled in the questionnaire in the waiting room, I had to concentrate to keep my writing hand steady. I tried to draw consolation from the fact that I could tick most of the boxes that made cancer less likely – healthy diet, never smoked, didn't drink much and so forth. But there wasn't a box for whether you'd had EBV for fifteen years, was there?

I studied the other women in the waiting room. Solemn faces, slumped shoulders. Nobody was talking. Statistically, a couple of us would probably have cancer. Apparently that was enough to silence the renowned Geordie chat.

Finally, it was my turn to enter the consulting room. I'll never forget that vast space painted in shades of grey, nor the silence as two consultants and one radiographer pored over my scans. The only sound was my own blood pounding. Then they disappeared into a side room for a private discussion, and I tried not to worry about what they couldn't talk about in front of me. I was left with a nurse and a medical student, the nurse trying to ease the strain with chit-chat, the medical student desperately pretending to take notes.

After a few minutes, the consultants strode back. They said my lump was caused by the breast changes involved in pregnancy, and nothing remotely to worry about. The enlarged glands in my armpit were probably related not to the lump but to my EBV.

Suddenly the world exploded into technicolour. I hadn't bounced out of a room as happily as that since my Cambridge interviews. Jon and I hugged in the waiting room, and that night I celebrated by taking an extra mouthful of water with my Aciclovir.

Lying in the bath afterwards, I couldn't stop grinning as I thought of my wonderful, cancer-free body. I would still be around to raise my child and write my book!

*

The following week, as Jon and I were taking Matty to the children's ward to get his latest fever and rigours (shakes) checked out, my mobile rang. It was Mum. Dad's routine blood test – something he had each year since his heart bypass – had set alarm bells ringing. He was told to go to the Freeman Hospital in Newcastle immediately.

Matty was discharged from hospital with a prescription for more antibiotics.

Dad was diagnosed with an aggressive form of leukaemia.

*

'Dear Lord, look at the state of you!' said Mum as I opened the door to her one drizzly winter afternoon.

'You're not looking so hot yourself.' She had lost weight. Her skin was grey. But what did I expect when she was spending eight hours a day in hospital with Dad while he went through chemotherapy? I couldn't even go with her to visit him because Dad wasn't allowed to see anyone who was suffering from an infection – and I was riddled with them.

'At least I'm clean,' said Mum. 'Will you please take off that dirty dressing gown and burn it?'

'This isn't dirt,' I said, looking down at a bright orange stain. 'It's Matty's regurgitated carrot puree.'

'Which of course makes all the difference,' said Mum. 'I'm going to the shops to buy you a new one.'

'There's no need. I told you already, I've got two others. This one is the—'

'Scruffy one, yes. I don't think anyone could doubt that.' She sighed. 'I guess I'll have to buy you a new scruffy one, then.'

'Do they sell those in shops?' I asked.

'You know what I mean.'

And with that, Mum was off before I could talk her round.

Twenty minutes later, she returned with a bulging carrier bag. I thanked her profusely and pulled out the cotton waffle dressing gown inside it.

I stared at it.

'You don't like it?' asked Mum.

'I love it!'

'Then what's the problem?'

I had to come clean; there's no keeping things from your psychiatrist mother. 'It's just, it's… white. I always thought that, when the time came to replace dressing gown number three, I would get something in a darker colour. Otherwise, it will end up looking like this one' – I gestured to the stains – 'in three minutes flat.'

Mum deflated. 'You're right.'

I realised I was sounding ungrateful when, in reality, I couldn't have felt more touched. To go to this effort when she had so many other things to occupy her thoughts? I shoved the dressing gown back into its bag and put it in the hallway. Then I returned to the porch and reached out to hug her.

She stepped backwards. 'Sweetheart, you can't hug me. If I catch your cold, I won't be allowed to see Dad.'

We stared at each other across the porch.

'I wish I could come with you to see him,' I murmured.

'I wish I could help out with that gorgeous boy of yours,' Mum replied, her voice cracking. Then she suddenly straightened and asked, 'Any laundry you want doing?'

I found some clothes to give her, and she left. Then, as I closed the door, I turned to pick up my new dressing gown and…

Oh, where was it? I knew I was brain fogged, but I was sure I had left it in the hall. When I checked there, though, I couldn't find it. I retraced my steps to the utility room, looking left and right across the kitchen. Still no dressing gown.

Then the penny dropped. *Mum, you sneak!*

I rang her on her mobile. 'Where are you?' I asked.

'Back at the shop.' I could hear her delight over the crackle on the line.

'With my dressing gown?'

'Yes!'

'How did you manage to slip the bag out without me noticing?'

'Good, aren't I?'

Soon, she was back on my doorstep, smiling as she returned the bag to me. I pulled out the dressing gown. It was fluffy. It was purple. It had bling. Three traits I would never have looked for in an item of clothing for myself. But my goodness, I loved it because it came from her. (And yes, OK, it got extra points for the fact that it wouldn't show the stains – I really am that boring.)

'Virtual hug?' I asked, extending my arms towards her.

'Virtual hug,' Mum agreed, copying the gesture.

*

My dad was dying. That's what they said. Due to the state of his heart, the doctors thought a stem cell transplant would probably kill him. Instead, he should enjoy his last six months of life. I was heartbroken, but I couldn't let Mum see that. Nor Matty. So, I kept my grieving to the dead of night, when I was alone in the kitchen downing antivirals.

Only once did my health improve sufficiently for me to visit Dad in hospital. His ward was strikingly fresh and sterile, but it had an unmistakable sombreness. Despite the mass of 'Get Well Soon' cards surrounding the patients' beds, there was an unspoken acceptance that this would only be possible for the minority. Dad filled us in on which of his new friends had died that week. We did our best to turn the chat towards lighter issues, then left when he needed to rest.

Later that day, someone coughed in the same postcode, and I came down with another cold. From then on, I mourned my father long distance.

The experience taught me that it's hard being unable to see loved ones when they are ill. Rationally, I knew the reasons why I couldn't visit Dad. But deep down I was a bit… hurt. His golf friends were allowed to see him. The priest was allowed to see him. And yet, his own daughter wasn't? It hit me then how my friends and family must have felt all the times I asked them to stay away. I understood why they complained about how little they saw me. Even when your mind knows why you must be apart, your soul can feel neglected.

Dad, meanwhile, was having revelations of his own. From things he tearfully said when I visited him, he had come to realise what it was like to be me. He would say to people: it was alright for him, he was well into his sixties and had had a good life. But this lonely world of feeling fuzzy and weak was the place I had inhabited since I was seventeen. A place where nobody understood you, and where you could do nothing except lie there and suffer while the world carried on without you.

*

Back at home, I became stuck once again in a viral rut. Jon had to take over with Matty more and more, so he wasn't getting much writing done. After much deliberation, we decided to put Matty in a nursery for a couple of sessions each week. Whilst I knew that it would be good for Matty to mix with other kids, I couldn't help feeling that I had 'failed'. I wasn't even able to look after my own child? How pathetic was that?

Whilst nursery provided Matty with new experiences, it also provided him with a string of new bugs – including chickenpox. I had never contracted the illness as a child because I was so ridiculously healthy (oh, the irony). Now, as I applied calamine lotion to Matty's lesions, I prayed I had unknowingly produced antibodies to the virus when my brother had been ill with it.

Yeah, right. A fortnight after Matty's first spot appeared, I was clearing the dining table when I started feeling faint. My head swirled, and strange sensations shot down my limbs. I hadn't felt this weird since I first contracted glandular fever. By midnight my temperature was forty degrees, and the following morning every square inch of my body was covered in spots.

One chickenpoxy morning, I put a pile of Duplo bricks and books down beside my bed and said to Matty, 'Sweetheart, Mummy's a bit poorly. Can you play here while I rest?'

Wishful thinking. The books kept Matty distracted for a whole five minutes, but he totally ignored the bricks – because why play with Duplo when there was a mummy to be clambered over? Soon, he was pulling at my covers and asking to see my belly button (he was totally obsessed with these, no idea why). As I pulled up my pyjama top to reveal my tummy, his gaze fixed on the spots there. He looked perplexed, then amused.

'Leper!' he shouted.

'Leper?' I repeated. I was amazed he knew the word. What sort of things were they teaching toddlers at nursery these days? So, I tested him. 'What's a leper?'

In response, he tottered out of my bedroom and turned left on the landing into his own. I heard books falling onto the floor from his bookcase, then he dashed back into my bedroom holding his animals board book. He hauled himself up and sat proudly on my chest, winding me in the process. You may have guessed what was coming next, but I had no idea.

Matty wrinkled his brow as he turned the pages, flicking past the pets and the farm animals until…

I laughed, finally understanding. 'Oh, you think Mummy looks like a leopard!'

He grinned and nodded.

'Well, maybe I do a bit,' I agreed. And I gave a little roar that startled him.

As I enfolded him in my arms, I didn't care about the chickenpox, or any other illness I would contract from him. He made everything special.

*

As Matty moved on to the next bug, I started to worry that I hadn't got him baptised. In the year or so since his birth, there hadn't been a weekend where both he and I had been well enough to attend church. Then Dad's leukaemia came along.

But miracles started happening. My dad went temporarily into remission just as a stem cell donor became available who was an excellent match for him. The cardiologist said he thought Dad might survive a transplant after all. Woo-hoo! Before, I'd been so resigned to Dad dying that I'd worked out what I would say at his funeral. Now, I could start thinking about a christening. It was such a sharp U-turn, it left my head spinning. But who cared so long as my dad would be around for longer?

We had to wait ages for both Matty and me to be infection-free, and therefore not a risk to Dad, whose immunity was still low after chemo. When that time came, Mum raced to the presbytery to make the arrangements. The priest had broken his ankle in a charity football match, but he understood the need for urgency. So, my parents, Jon, Matty and I gathered in his dining room, where he wobbled about on crutches and baptised Matty in what looked suspiciously like a mixing bowl. Afterwards, I read a poem, and Matty marked the occasion with an impromptu rendition of 'Twinkle Twinkle Little Star' during the prayers.

The star of the show, though, was my dad. His hair was starting to grow back after the chemo, and the rays of sunlight reflecting off it made him look almost ethereal. I'd chosen my parents as godparents, primarily so no one else needed to come to the christening (in case they gave Dad a bug). But as I watched him read from the Bible, I realised I couldn't have picked a more noble godfather for Matty. Dad is the kindest and most sincere person I know, and he never lost his faith through his illness even as others died around him. I hoped his tale would have a happy ever after.

Sure enough, Dad survived his bone marrow transplant and was back on the golf course a few months later. I learnt from his ordeal that there are worse illnesses than ME/CFS, but I also learnt that there are wonderful individuals in the world. My dad's stem cell donor saved his life – and he didn't even know him. Sometimes, when others are dismissive or bigoted about ME/CFS, it can make you think people are heartless. But then a stranger gives part of himself to another stranger, like Dad's donor did, and you realise that there are healthy people out there who understand the hardships of others and want to help them. It lifts the soul. It is totally inspiring. Thank you, whoever you are. Thank you.

Chapter 18

I would soon be thirty-four, which meant I had been ill for half my life. Matty's health was improving, and so was mine now that he was at nursery. Finally, I had a little leftover health to spend on myself. So, I got my hair done, reminded myself how to drive, even treated myself to a trip to the dentist. I know, I know, I really know how to spoil myself.

I hadn't been well enough to go to a dentist for over a decade, so I was dreading what problems she might discover. As I was raised towards the bright light, I gripped the arms of the chair. Fortunately, my teeth were in good shape apart from a wisdom tooth that needed extracting. The dentist gave me an injection and set about removing it. I really felt like I was being fixed, both emotionally and physically.

Then the tooth shattered, sending bits of enamel flying across the room, and exposing the roots. I was told that I would need dental surgery at another clinic to remove what remained.

A day or two later, I was in the clinic's waiting room with Jon and Matty. The dentist was running late, so Matty found novel ways of entertaining himself, like climbing into the window display and almost impaling his hand on a yucca.

As I dragged him back to his chair, a burly man came out clutching his cheek and holding back tears. It did not bode well.

'Oh, wisdom teeth roots are easy!' the dentist reassured me when I entered the treatment room. 'Three minutes, max.'

But after an hour of drilling and blood-vacuuming, not to mention the ministrations of a myriad of tools that should never go near someone's mouth, the roots remained in place. Further X-rays confirmed that they were trapped beneath the adjacent tooth. There was only one solution: the dentist would have to sew me back up and simply hope things settled down of their own accord. Otherwise, I would need a trip to hospital for surgery.

'You know,' said the dentist, 'things like this only happen about once a year. You're my Unlucky Patient of the Year!' She said it with such exuberance, I half expected her to whip out a rosette and pin it to my blood-spattered collar.

On the way back to the car, I relayed all this to Jon.

'It had to be you, didn't it?' he grumbled. 'When are you going to catch a break?'

When I rang Mum, she said much the same thing: 'Lily, you are officially the most unfortunate young woman I have ever met.'

So, I decided to call Caja next. She always knew how to cheer me up.

'There should be some law about how much misfortune one person can have in their lifetime,' she said. 'It's just not right!'

Unsure how to respond, I sat there holding the phone in one hand and massaging my swollen jaw with the other.

'All I can think,' Caja went on, 'is that your life is about to turn around in a big way. Maybe you'll never have another relapse. And Jon will get a major book deal. And Matty will grow into the loveliest boy ever. Otherwise, life is just not fair.'

I appreciated her empathy, but I didn't share her viewpoint, nor that of Jon and Mum. OK, my cheek was now so distended it made my face look lopsided. Everyone stared at me as I walked down the street. But my swelling would only be temporary. What about all the people out there with permanent disfigurements? What must life be like for them? Having a wonky face made me realise how many different forms of disability there were, and I resolved always to try to appreciate others' problems. If not, what right did I have to expect people to understand mine?

I remember a conversation I had around that time with a Scottish chap in the immunology department of my hospital in Newcastle. I was waiting to be called in for a blood test when, out of the blue, the man on the next seat leaned over and posed me a question: who is really living? The people with chronic ill health like us, or the healthy people rushing around oblivious to how good they have it?

I understood what he was getting at. In his eyes I saw not suffering, but the joy that comes when the suffering subsides. I felt a kinship with this middle-aged guy. And I knew, just as he will have done, that we belonged to the same club. I don't mean a shitty-immune-system club. I mean, we were the survivors who had seen the world from both sides and could now appreciate every morsel of life we were given. We weren't affected as much by the minor annoyances that can get other people down. We were too busy appreciating the wonderful thing that it is to be alive. It's the best club ever.

*

Eventually, my tooth sorted itself out, and I was able to turn my attention to the next item on my imaginary to-do list: whether I should try for a second child. I had always wanted two children. My dream family consisted of an older boy and a younger girl, but was I really capable of raising another child? Matty was now a robust two-and-a-half-year-old, and my own health was the best it had been for seventeen years. Yet, I had relapsed badly when I had Matty, and only started fighting the EBV once we increased his hours at nursery. Another baby now could catapult me back to square one.

After lengthy chats with Jon, we decided to quit while we were ahead and sell our baby equipment at the next National Childbirth Trust sale before we could change our minds.

As fate would have it, the sale was being held at my old school – the one I'd been in when I fell ill all those years ago. In the run-up to the event, I didn't think about the significance of that. But as Jon parked the car in the school's courtyard, I felt overcome with loss. This was the courtyard that I wrote about earlier in this book: the one where I'd told the teacher I was fine to ski. To my left I could see the science block where I had castrated the rat and spilt ink over my botany practical.

This was where my story began. But this was also where things had started to go wrong.

Jon was unloading the travel cot, oblivious to my distress. 'Where do I take this?' he asked.

'To the dining hall,' I replied, unclipping Matty from his car seat. 'I'm glad we're going there, actually. There's something I want to show you.'

We headed past the site of the former tuck shop, then around the back of the laboratories. It was a route I had walked a thousand times before, in the days when my head was full of hope and science. Inside, there were women everywhere, cooing over each other's babies in slings. The dining hall was bustling with people setting out their sale items and eyeing up everyone else's. Matty pulled at my arm and pointed towards a side room where the toys were being laid out. He'd already spotted a farm set and tractor.

'Wait,' I said, restraining him. 'There's something I need to show Daddy first.' I turned to Jon. 'See these?' I said, gesturing to the wooden award boards on the walls. People who had won academic prizes at school were listed here. 'Try and find me on them.'

Jon looked up. 'It must have been for chemistry,' he mused, 'so... there you are. Twice!'

'Yes, but one time was shared. Does it count if you share a prize?'

'Absolutely.' He continued to scan the boards. 'There you are again for biology. And what the hell is "recitations"?'

'Ah, there's a story there. My boyfriend at the time was entering the poetry reading competition, and I offered to help him prepare. But he got in such a huff, he started mouthing off at me, saying what would I know about poetry? So, at the last minute I tracked down the teacher in charge and asked if I could enter.'

'And you won?'

'Yes.' (That one was shared too.) 'Sometimes you have to prove a point, don't you? But I'm not like that any more.'

'Of course not,' muttered Jon.

'What I mean is, I now know there are ways of making your point that don't involve going into battle over it.'

I thought back to my school days when I felt I'd had something to prove to the doubters. If I had my time again,

I would handle things differently. We were all just teenagers trying to find our place in the world. The other girls couldn't understand my experiences or priorities any more than I could theirs. But we all grow up and gain perspective. I have learnt that understanding others is more important than showing your own worth.

I looked around again, soaking up the ambience of my former life. It had been fifteen years since I had eaten in these halls, but the memories still tugged at me in a way I couldn't control. Like the time I piled my dinner tray high with chips, cheese, sponge pudding and custard after a particularly gruelling hockey match. Needless to say, my diet has improved along with my attitude.

I left Matty with Jon and went outside again to sort out what I was feeling. It had all become too much. The realisation that my chance at a science career was over, and that I wasn't up to having another baby, had left me feeling… empty. But the recognition that I was now happy with who I had become was starting to fill the void.

Then, like an angel materialising, Mum appeared in front of me. She put her arm around me.

'Thought you might need some support,' she said.

'With the sale?'

'With your emotions.'

'Thank you.' I sniffed. 'I mean, I knew I'd find it hard getting rid of the baby gear, but I hadn't considered how I would feel seeing the prize boards and the labs.'

'Well, I did consider it,' Mum said. 'That's why I came.' She rooted through a pocket before handing me… a cloth.

'Tell me that's not another relic,' I said, only half joking.

'It's a clean hanky, love.'

It smelt of Persil washing powder, and that reminded me of freshly washed school uniforms, and gym kits, and days when I had had the health to do whatever I wanted.

We sat for a while on the wall outside the music department, each alone with our thoughts.

'Do you think it's true what they say?' I asked at last. 'That you don't get what you want in life, but you get what you need?'

She didn't reply, but I already had my own answer. I had come full circle in school that day. I had relived all that loss and realised I still felt fulfilled. So yes, it was true for me.

'Should I walk up the steps to the chapel?' I asked Mum. 'Just to show how much better I am now?'

'No,' she said in her best headmistress voice. 'I think you should go home and rest.'

*

I hit the health books afresh, determined to become the strongest mother I could be. I hadn't been well enough to read properly for years, and somehow Matty's toddler books weren't stretching me.

I read meditation books by Buddhists, guides on happiness, pieces on epigenetics... Epigenetics is the study of gene expression. Put simply, you are born with a particular set of genes, but the extent to which those genes are active can be influenced by how you live. Your diet, your outlook, how many toxins you take in: all of these and more can have a bearing on your condition. So even if you find yourself lumped with an illness, your prognosis is not set in stone.

Changing your lifestyle isn't easy, and it comes with no

written guarantee – I have the gradually emptying beds on my dad's cancer ward to demonstrate that. But for people whose illness isn't terminal, at least it's a start.

Of course, holistic health isn't just about looking after the mind and body – the soul has to be addressed too. Whatever the explanation for the 'otherworldly' experiences I described earlier in this book – for example, the bedtime column of light and the sensation of a presence at my side on the postbox walk – they taught me not to forget the importance of spirituality. Spirituality means something different to every person, but whether you believe in someone up there or not, please don't forget your connectedness with others. I think I needed to be ill to fully feel that.

While absorbing myself in books on health, I had another realisation: the curious scientist was still inside me and would always be, because that's who I am. It didn't matter to me any more that I wouldn't have a degree to prove it.

By now, Jon had sent his book off to literary agents. One morning, he poked his head around the bedroom door and said, 'You're not going to believe this email!'

It was from an agent's reader, checking Jon hadn't signed to anyone else yet. The next day there was an email from the agent himself, offering representation. We were delirious. We were incredulous. We were… well, pretty drunk to be honest after all the champagne we got through.

A handful of international book deals followed, meaning Jon had finally found fulfilment. Matty, meanwhile, was as hyper as ever, but he was blossoming into a loyal and caring young boy. He was now nearing the end of his time at nursery, and Jon and I decided to move house again so we could be close to his primary school. All the lugging and clearing was a relapse waiting to happen, but fortunately Jon's parents spared me from that fate by helping with the hard graft. I wouldn't have survived the move without them.

I suspect that Jon's mother still felt she was missing out on Matty's life, but at this point, even our infrequent get-togethers were stretching my health to breaking point. While venting my frustrations in my diary one day, I thought, *why am I writing this down instead of explaining it to people's faces?* So, with a bit of help from Jon, I let comments slip to my in-laws about my feelings and limitations.

The following Christmas, having fought a fever to make the trip down to Nottingham, Jon's mum was talking to me about another of her grandsons, who has autism. She said, 'The thing is, I think all the obstacles he has had to overcome are going to make him stronger. Because that's what your illness has done for you, hasn't it, Lily?' And she smiled at me with such warmth that I nearly melted.

When we were leaving a few days later, car filled to the roof with duvets, pillows and Christmas presents, the vehicle was already in reverse when Jon's mum rushed out of her house and tapped on my window. I buzzed it down.

'I just wanted to say, thank you for coming,' she said. 'I know it will have taken a lot out of you, and I hope it doesn't set you back too far.'

I am so grateful for her words. It was a 'Eureka!' moment for me, because it showed that people would come to understand this illness if I explained it fully.

Caja's prophecy about things turning around in my life was coming true. Now I just had to get well enough to finish this book. I drew up an immune-boosting regime of supplements and happy thoughts and put my headphones on for some epigenetic visualisations. As you do.

*

In the summer before Matty started school, I was snatching a lie-down in the lounge when he raced up and pressed his face against mine.

'Let's play pirates!' he said, taking my hand and trying to haul me off the sofa. I pulled him in for a cuddle instead. He yielded for a whole two seconds, then begged, 'Now pirates! Pleeeeeease!'

'What do we have to do?' I asked warily.

'We run round and pretend we're pirates!'

'I'm sorry, sweetheart. I'm not sure Mummy is up to running.'

'Then Mummy can *walk* around and pretend she's a pirate,' he said matter-of-factly. 'And I'll run extra.'

I laughed but felt powerless. My glands were already the size of marbles, but how could I tell him that walking around might be enough to tip me into a full relapse? I needed a plan. I was becoming adept at tailoring the activity levels of games so that I didn't damage my health.

After a think I said, 'OK, but I'm the naughty pirate.'

I watched his face, waiting to see if he would take the bait. He did.

'Then walk the plank!' he said.

Next thing I knew, I was being led along one of our oak floorboards with a plastic cutlass poking my bottom. I feigned falling into the sea and dying. After Matty had finished giggling he said, 'Mummy, you can get up now.'

'No, I can't. The sharks have injured me badly. In fact, I think I might be dead.' I planned to milk this lie-down for all it was worth.

'No, Mummy, you're still alive. And we're rescuing you from the sea.'

Not if I had anything to say about it. 'But a shark has just eaten my legs! I'll definitely need to stay here.'

He frowned while he thought this over. 'Well OK, but only for a little bit. There's lots of work to do.'

'Like what?'

'Like sorting out the treasure.'

'I can do that!' I said, figuring that as long as I showed willing, I could stay horizontal throughout.

So Matty ran upstairs to fetch his little treasure chests, then tipped out all of the plastic coins, sequins and fake gems. As he started arranging them into piles, he said, 'I like sorting things.'

'Me too,' I replied. 'I used to do a lot of that when I was little.'

'Did you run round lots too?'

'No. I mean, I liked to run. But I also liked being still sometimes.'

He looked at me as if the word 'still' was from a foreign language. 'But we like the same things now, don't we? Like sorting things.'

'Like sorting things,' I agreed.

'And playing pirates.'

'Er, yeah. That too.'

And we talked about other things we enjoyed, while I let the happy hormones flow through me, washing away painful memories of my past.

*

One day, Matty arrived home covered in mud after a trip to Durham University's Botanic Garden with Jon, so I ran a bath for him. He played with his Playmobil while we waited for the tub to fill; he had a family of plastic characters in a speedboat, jetting off towards the tub. When the taps were turned off, he climbed into the bath with his boatful of figures, leaving behind a single brown-haired Playmobil lady on the floor.

'Don't forget this one,' I told Matty, picking her up. 'She's been left behind.'

'No, that's the mummy,' he said dismissively. 'She doesn't come out to have fun. She stays behind to rest.' And he took her out of my hand before placing her back down on the floor. On her front. Just as I lie in bed.

I felt crushed. I had never discussed my illness with Matty before, but it seemed my attempts to hide it from him had failed. Because of my condition, taking him out had always been the privilege of his dad and grandparents. If I wanted him to stop seeing me like that brown-haired Playmobil lady, then things would have to change.

Later, I talked it through with Jon, and we agreed to get out more as a family – to the countryside, just the three of us, every weekend I was able to pull some clothes on.

I've recently treated myself to a slide show of old photos on the computer to remind myself of the places we went: the derelict castles of Northumberland, the ruins of Hadrian's Wall. As I view the pictures of us paddling in the North Sea, buckets in hands, I can still feel the icy air on my face. Matty's rosy cheek is squashed into my white and blobby one, the pair of us radiating happiness. After nearly two decades of illness, I was finally able to get out and enjoy life with the people I loved the most.

Of course, 'getting out' and 'enjoying life' mean something different to me than they do to a healthy person. Nowadays, most of my time is spent stress-testing benches as I walk the fine line between health and relapse. But for years, Matty did not realise that my ill health was the reason why his dad took off with him to play on the zip-wire or find the next clue in the trail. All that mattered to him was that the three of us were together.

That's how I manage my life now: I use my moments of health to do what is important. ME/CFS is not an illness that you 'beat'; you either bend with it, or you break. I get up each morning, take my elderberry, and do the best I can with the health that I've been granted for that day. My experiences have made me see life through a clearer lens, and that is something I am truly grateful for.

Of course, most medics advise that ME/CFS sufferers adopt this strategy of managing their lifestyle, but that approach is only feasible once a patient's health has progressed to a certain level. Adjusting your mindset to *limited* health is comparatively easy once you have passed the hurdle of being bedbound. However, getting past the bedbound stage usually needs medical attention. Cracking this illness is teamwork.

I realise that not every case of ME/CFS will be due to EBV, but with every draft of this book, I have found more up-to-date research suggesting it is the culprit in a large proportion of cases. In 2014, a paper published in *PLOS One* showed that up to seventy-six per cent of the four hundred or so ME/CFS patients in the study had a reduced ability to control their EBV – like me.[a] At the end of 2021, there was a brilliant paper published suggesting that my subgroup of ME/CFS has an 'acquired immunodeficiency after EBV infection'.[b] Its proposed mechanisms would explain just about everything that has happened to me. This paper explores possible genetic tests and future treatments... so there is hope of progress, as long as the research continues.

I wrote this book long before the coronavirus pandemic, but as I edit it, it is long Covid that is grabbing the headlines. The similarities in symptoms between ME/CFS and long Covid – from brain fog to joint pains – are striking. 'This new cohort of [long Covid] patients... should not have to suffer the same mistakes that have been inflicted on people with ME/CFS,' said Dr Charles Shepherd in a letter to the BMJ.[c] This gives me confidence that the lessons learnt from the mismanagement of ME/CFS will ultimately help sufferers of long Covid. Looking online now, it is clear that many researchers of both ME/CFS and long Covid believe this is the case, and that the research into the overlap between these two conditions will improve the understanding of both.

In my case, I had, and still suffer from, the effects of EBV, and it has taken a whole book to explain how my illness was untangled. But I am one of the lucky ones: I got my answers. There are over a million ME/CFS sufferers out there who don't have that privilege. I hope that my story, combined with emerging research, will persuade a few uncertain medics that cases like mine need to be investigated. It is inappropriate to send the patient away just with a label of ME/CFS, and no guidance on how to treat it. When Sajid Javid was health secretary, he pledged more research to tackle the condition, after a relative was diagnosed with it. He described the attitude of some doctors as follows: 'When you can't find out what the true cause is, let's just call it ME/CFS – a sort of convenient bucket – and let's just leave [them] in that bucket.'[tl] He promised radical action, but will the present and future health secretaries measure up to that pledge?

In my prologue, I mentioned the range of alternative names for ME/CFS. Personally, I regard my illness as chronic EBV. However, I don't mind if people call it that, or ME/CFS, or something else, as long as they understand that it is a form of immune dysregulation – resulting in frequent glandular fever relapses and a susceptibility to other infections – and not tiredness! I suspect that the naming of the illness will always be a contentious issue, but I can't help thinking that the gravity of the condition would be better understood if we stopped calling it fatigue.

*

One afternoon, after Matty had started primary school, I put my once-again grubby four-year-old in the bath and handed him the bath crayons while I sorted out the laundry. I was gathering together a pile of clothing when I heard a splash.

'Oh no!' Matty said. 'Mummy, help!'

'What is it?'

'I need the light pink, but it fell in the water. I can't find it.'

The bath water was opaque from the skin-friendly bath oil I use, so I couldn't see anything either. 'Sweetheart, can you not just use the other pink instead?'

'This one?' he asked, holding up the darker pink crayon.

'Yes.'

He shook his head. 'It's too dark.'

'For what? What are you drawing?'

'Your face.'

Uh oh, I thought, fearing another Playmobil moment. I dropped the pile of clothes I was holding and knelt by the bath to look at the sketches he had drawn on the side of it. I recognised Jon from his bright blue eyes. Along from him was a grinning self-portrait of Matty. He had even drawn the bit of his hair that sticks up at the front.

'But you used the darker pink crayon to draw yours and Daddy's faces, so why don't you use it for mine?'

'Because you're whiter, Mummy.'

He was alluding to the pallor that comes with my illness, but I had thought I had a bit more colour in my cheeks these days. 'I'm paler than you and Daddy?' I enquired. The two of them have the sort of complexion that turns lobster when they blink at the sun.

'Yes! Look in the mirror, Mummy!'

I studied my reflection and he was right: I did have my ghoulish appearance back. The one that comes just before my glands start to enlarge.

Matty's expression was solemn. 'That's why I need the *light* pink,' he said. 'I want it perfect.'

I knew how he felt. As a teenager, I had been so fixed on details that it used to hurt me if I lost a mark in an exam. Then there was the time I broke a finger playing netball, and the worst thing was not the pain but the fact that it spoiled my handwriting. But standing in the bathroom with Matty, I realised that none of that stuff mattered to me any more. I had learnt the hard way that there is no such thing as perfection; you have to make the best of what you've been given in life and find happiness in the imperfections.

I was wondering how to explain this to a four-year-old when Matty declared he had come up with a solution: he would not colour me in at all, leaving my face the white of the bath. And to think I'd been worried about being light pink. Not knowing what to say, I kissed him on the forehead instead.

'Yuck,' he said.

A few minutes later, an excited yelp informed me that he had found the pale pink crayon after all, stuck under the bathmat. Thrilled, he finished our family portrait: Daddy, Matty and ghostly Mummy. He looked at it thoughtfully.

'Mummy,' he said. 'Why do the boys in my class like their daddies more than their mummies?'

'Do they?'

'All the boys I asked. But I love you the same. Daddy is more fun to play with...'

Cheers, I thought.

'But you're more...' He stopped. 'You're like...'

I stared at him, curious how the sentence would end. How *did* my perfectionist son view his chronically ill mother?

As he struggled to find the right words, he waved his tiny hands like a baby bird trying to take off. It was so cute I had to stop myself laughing. Then he grinned and said, 'You're a superhero!' And he picked up the yellow crayon and drew a smiley sun on the tiles above our heads.

I blinked back tears. His words showed that my disabilities didn't matter so long as I was there for him. But a superhero? I smiled as I imagined myself in big pants and a cape.

'Just a very pale one?' I said.

'Just a very pale one,' he agreed.

References

Prologue

a. Munn S E. More than defeatism greets patients with ME. *BMJ* 2010;340:c1179.

b. Williams T. Chronic Fatigue: NHS faces 'post coronavirus tsunami' as survivors are struck by ME, docs warn. *The Sun*. 25 June, 2020. Accessed January 18, 2022. https://www.thesun.co.uk/news/11951847/nhs-post-coronavirus-tsunami-survivors-struck-by-me.

c. Williams F M K, Muirhead N, Pariante C. Covid-19 and chronic fatigue. *BMJ* 2020;370:m2922.

Chapter 14

a. Jones J F, Ray C G, Minnich L L, Hicks M J, Kibler R, Lucas D O. Evidence for active Epstein-Barr virus infection in patients with persistent, unexplained illnesses: elevated anti-early antigen antibodies. *Ann Intern Med*. 1985;102(1):1-7.

Chapter 15

a. Kimura H, Morishima T, Kanegane H, et al. Prognostic factors for chronic active Epstein-Barr virus infection. *J Infect Dis*. 2003;187(4):527-533.

Chapter 18

a. Loebel M, Strohschein K, Giannini C, et al. Deficient EBV-

specific B- and T-cell response in patients with chronic fatigue syndrome. *PLOS ONE.* 2014;9(1):e85387.
b. Ruiz-Pablos M, Paiva B, Montero-Mateo R, Garcia N, Zabaleta A. Epstein-Barr Virus and the Origin of Myalgic Encephalomyelitis or Chronic Fatigue Syndrome. *Front Immunol.* 2021;12:656797.
c. Shepherd C B. Charities, patients, and researchers are working together to find the cause and effective treatments for ME/CFS. *BMJ* 2021;374:n1854.
d. Torjesen I. Health secretary pledges more ME/CFS research as he reveals that relative has condition. *BMJ* 2022;377:o1341.

Books

In case any of the books I mentioned sparked an interest, here are further details:

Reader's Digest. *Foods That Harm, Foods That Heal: An A-Z Guide to Safe and Healthy Eating.* Reader's Digest; 1996.

Loblay R, Soutter V, Swain A. *Friendly Food: The Essential Guide to Avoiding Allergies, Additives and Problem Chemicals.* Murdoch Books; 2004.

Rainer T. *Your Life as Story: Discovering the 'New Autobiography' and Writing Memoir as Literature.* Tarcher/Putnam,US; 1998.

Hamilton R, Heap S. *Let's Take Over The Nursery!* Bloomsbury Publishing PLC; 2007.

Shepherd C. *Living With M.E.: The Chronic/Post-Viral Fatigue Syndrome.* Vermilion; 1999.